DIET for the
SPORTS-MINDED MALE ©

Using Sports Strategies to Lose Weight and Gain Health

DIET for the
SPORTS-MINDED MALE ©

Using Sports Strategies to Lose Weight and Gain Health

Ray Burigo, MS, RD, CISSN, CPT

ACKNOWLEDGMENTS

I would like to give special thanks to Libby for all her help and encouragement. I would also like to acknowledge five of my best friends: Sebastian, Piper, Santiago, Carlotta, and Henri.

DISCLAIMER

This publication contains the opinions and ideas of the author. It is intended to provide informative information on the subject of weight loss and nutrition and not for the purpose of rendering medical, health, or any other kind of personal services. The reader should consult his (or her) medical, health, or other competent professional before adopting any suggestions found in this book.

The author and publisher specifically disclaim all responsibility for any liability, loss, or risk, personal or otherwise, which is incurred as a consequence, directly or indirectly, of the use and application of any of the contents of the book.

CONTENTS

Preface:
Why Sports-Minded Males?

In sports, a good game plan is useless without players capable of executing the plan. And the same holds true for dieting. A healthy diet plan is also useless without dieters capable of following the diet. I have never understood why diets are constantly being scrutinized for their worthiness, while the worthiness of the dieter is never considered. The way I see it, there is not a lack of qualified diets, but rather a lack of qualified dieters. That's why I have written a diet specifically for a group that is qualified—sports-minded males. It is my opinion that sports-minded males have everything it takes to achieve the long-term dietary success that has eluded 80 percent of dieters.[1]

On the surface, the typical American male may not appear to be a prime candidate for dietary success. In fact, most guys scoff at the idea of dieting. But who can blame them? Like most Americans, they have become discouraged and confused with the entire notion of dieting. All their efforts have been wasted on diets that have been too difficult to follow, too tasteless, or too ridiculous to mention. Besides, guys don't like being told what to do, and they especially don't like being told what to eat. What they need is a legitimate diet written specifically for them. And now they have it.

---

1. Rena R. Wing, and James O. Hill, *Successful Weight Maintenance*. Annual Review of Nutrition, 2001, vol. **21**: pp. 323–341.

Introduction:
The Winning Formula

First, I would like to clarify what I mean by the term "diet." This book uses the term diet in the true sense of the word. A diet, by definition, is a person's normal or habitual way of eating. It is not what is commonly referred to as a diet which is typically a neurotic attempt to lose a few pounds by starving yourself or giving up carbohydrates while exercising like a madman. That's not what this diet is about. The goal of this diet is to improve your normal way of eating (diet), for the rest of your life, in a rational, step-by-step fashion. The idea is to create a plan that enables you to eat intelligently all of the time and not just when you get the urge to drop a few pounds. In other words, the goal is to do this "dieting thing" right, for once and for all.

Diet for the Sports-Minded Male was written to be short, simple, and to the point. I feel that the subject of dieting has become overly complicated. There seems to be hundreds of theories as to the best way to lose weight. These theories become popular because it appears more promising and hopeful for the dieters if their weight problem has something to do with their blood type, hormones, glycemic index, or with them not eating the precise combination of macronutrients. Sure, some of these theories play a role, but they do not address the primary problem for most dieters. I say enough already with the theories. We are going to keep this nice and simple. We are going to start with the premise that you eat too much and work from there. There is no need to get more complicated than that. I am not trying to be funny or overly simplistic or tell you something that you already know. What I'm trying to do is to put things in the proper perspective. The goal of this book is to get you back in shape by focusing on the most important issues, not to distract you with another half-baked theory.

This book will be using sports analogies, strategies, and motivational techniques to transform dieting into an invigorating challenge similar to that of training for a sport. The same time-tested principles that you already know and understand can now be used to get you back into shape. Sports strategies will be used because they work and you understand them. Think about it; athletes keep getting better and better, while dieters continue to struggle. So why not use the methods that have worked? The premise is quite simple; if you understand what it takes to win at sports, then you have what it takes to be successful at dieting.

THE GAME PLAN

Diet for the Sports-Minded Male mimics a typical sports season complete with a training camp and an off-season. Specific dieting skills are practiced during training camp, one at a time. After proper preparation, the season begins and you will then attempt to put it all together. This is followed by the well deserved off-season when you can relax and enjoy your accomplishments while restoring motivation for the following season. The off-season dispels the notion that going off a diet should somehow be considered a failure. The only failure is not recognizing the natural ebb and flow of life. There is a time to lose, a time to gain, and a time to remain the same. That's life; we are not going to fight it.

As in sports, a perfect blend of seriousness and play is encouraged. You will be put at ease as you follow the trials and tribulations of the book's three fictional characters—Fast-Food Freddy, Snack-Happy Steve, and Duck-Hook Harry, for an entire dieting season. These characters are composites of the many men I have counseled over the past twenty-one years. They will voice the concerns of most guys, relieving any doubt as to the proper way to proceed. To simplify matters even more, extensive lists of food choices will be given, answering the number one question of most guys — "So, what can I eat?" Food choices will be ranked as Gold, Silver, Bronze, or Zero-Value, making it possible for you to progress at your own realistic pace.

In addition, *Diet for the Sports-Minded Male* provides a system of accountability. In sports, a score kept so all can plainly see who are winning or losing. This diet will provide scorecards, enabling you to examine your diet like the back of a baseball card. Simple calculations make it easy to determine whether your diet is adhering to the recommendations for twelve key nutritional categories.

You will also be learning how to make food choices all by yourself. Nobody will be telling you exactly what to eat as if you were ten years old. You will be learning not only what to eat but also how to make the transition to a healthier lifestyle.

In summary, this book is not about trying to invent some new magical way of eating. There isn't any. This is about you, your health, and the stone-cold facts about nutrition. This is not about following my diet or anybody else's. This is going to be *your* diet. We are going to make improvements to your current diet one meal at a time, at your own pace. Only you will be able to choose what changes you are capable of making, what changes you want to make, and at what pace you want to make them. I'll help by providing the game plan, but you'll be doing the work. I truly believe that sport-minded males can do anything that they set their minds to do. So let's do it!

Chapter 1:
The Concept of Seasons

In sports, a season is designed according to the natural ebb and flow of life. Each season includes a time of preparation (training camp), a time to test what you have learned (season), and a period of contemplation, restoration, and relaxation (off-season).

Diet for the Sports-Minded Male will incorporate the concept of a season by implementing what will be called a "dieting cycle." Similar to a sports season, a dieting cycle will begin with a training camp, followed by the season, and then ending with the all-important off-season. A dieting cycle is roughly four months long, allowing for three dieting cycles per year.

The first cycle starts in January with its off-season in April. The training camp of cycle two begins in May getting you ready for the summer. The off-season of the second cycle is in August, which is a good time to kick back, relax, and enjoy the end of the summer. The training camp of cycle three begins in September with the off-season coinciding with the holidays. The three cycles equal forty-eight weeks leaving four wild-card weeks that you can add to any of the cycles during the course of the year. For example, you may be doing very well losing weight during a particular training camp and wish to continue for another week or two. Or perhaps you may not be ready to begin a new training camp and elect to prolong your off-season a bit longer. The choice will be yours.

Over the years I have found that many sports-minded males get the urge to lose weight and get into better shape about three times a year. These urges normally surface at the start of a new year, during the spring, and again in the fall. The dieting cycles will give these natural urges some well-needed structure so that motivation and progress can be sustained throughout the year. With three dieting cycles per year, you will have plenty of opportunities to improve. There is absolutely no need to turn your world upside down in a frantic quest to drop a few quick pounds. The cultivation of patience is probably a new dieting concept for many to digest, and it may take some time to get used to. Most of us are accustomed to going all-out until we drop. Most of us have learned that it doesn't work. So please, don't try to go from pig to perfect overnight. To master a sport takes multiple seasons. The same realistic approach is needed for dieting.

TRAINING CAMP—WEEKS 1-4 (QUALITY CONTROL)

Another concept borrowed from the world of sports is the training camp. In all sports, you just don't run out onto the field and start playing. Many hours of practice are needed before a player actually competes in a game. The fundamentals of each sport are first practiced individually before attempting to put it all together in game conditions. For the sport of basketball, the skills of shooting, passing, dribbling, and defense are practiced endlessly before the season ever starts. Baseball has its own group of fundamentals, such as hitting, fielding, bunting, and throwing. And we are all aware that you don't dare go near a golf course without first spending countless hours at the driving range.

Bobby Knight once said that the will to win isn't nearly as important as the will to prepare to win. Everyone has the will to win on game day, but not everyone has the will to prepare for it. Likewise, the will to get into shape isn't nearly as important as the will to prepare to get into shape. Most sports-minded males have a tremendous will to get into shape, but often, the preparation is lacking. *Diet for the Sports-Minded Male* will rectify this oversight by instituting a training camp in the beginning of every dieting cycle.

Each dieting cycle begins with a training camp that is eight weeks long. During the first four weeks we will be improving the quality of our food choices one meal at a time. During these first four weeks we will not be overly concerned with calorie restriction or weight loss. The main strategy of this diet is not to try to do everything at once. Improving the quality of the foods you are eating is a sufficient first step. You will also be more likely to alter or change your food choices if you are not being restricted to eating smaller amounts. The improved food choices made during this period will automatically improve the nutrient content and quality of your diet. Chances are also good that you will automatically be eating fewer calories and losing weight simply by improving your food choices and by continually focusing on what you are eating. The cumulative effects of constant awareness of your food choices will have a dramatic effect on your health.

Improvements to your diet will be made one meal at a time. During week one of training camp you will be making improvements to your breakfast and morning snack. Week two will follow by making better selections for your lunch and afternoon snack. Week three continues with improvements for your dinner/dessert and evening snack. The improvements made during the first three weeks will then be sustained for the fourth week and the upcoming season.

TRAINING CAMP—WEEKS 5-8 (QUANTITY CONTROL)

The final four weeks of training camp are focused on quantity control (calorie restriction). Calorie restriction is a major pain in the ass and I don't know of anyone who enjoys it. But that's what is needed in order to lose body fat. Fortunately, calorie restriction is required for only four weeks at a time, three times per year.

The maximum weight loss for one week is about two pounds. One pound can be expected from the restriction of five hundred calories per day for one week. The other pound comes from the three thousand five hundred calories burned through exercise for the week. Be careful not to base your dietary success solely on weight loss. People gain and lose weight at different rates. You know your body better than anyone, so be realistic. Remember, you are trying to do this "dieting thing" right for once and for all. The goal is not just lose a few pounds for the hundredth time, only to gain them right back; it is to keep those pounds off, by taking control of your eating for the rest of your life.

THE SEASON

As in sports, the season is ready to start at the end of training camp. The season is the time that puts all of your recent dietary changes to the test—when you see how many of the things that were practiced during training camp can actually be continued during your normal everyday life. Our goal is to continue the progress made during training camp into the season. What you eat during this time period of four weeks can actually be considered *your* diet. This time period is really the best indicator of how well you are doing. Each training camp gives you the opportunity to improve your diet a little bit at a time. And each subsequent season gives you the opportunity to make those improvements a normal part of your life.

THE OFF-SEASON

Having an off-season changes the entire foundation of dieting. Obsessively fretting over food choices every day of the year is not normal. This obsession with food creates a formidable strain that is usually relieved by overeating. Paradoxically, the need to overeat diminishes when you begin to cut yourself some slack. This is your chance to sit back and reassess the completed season. The off-season is a planned celebration for a job well done. This is in direct contrast to the guilt-ridden pig-outs that usually follow a failed diet. This downtime is critical for the rejuvenation of energy and motivation for the next season, creating a pattern that can be continued for the rest of your life.

DEFENSE

During the off-season you will have to play defense. Defense wins games. This is true in sports, and it's true for dieting. Let me explain what I mean by this. In the game of dieting, being on offensive is comparable to the times that you are watching what you eat and trying to lose some weight. In other words, being on offense means having a good dieting day. These good days are the cornerstone of most diets. But the part of a diet that is often overlooked is the defensive side of dieting. By defense, I mean the effort to control overeating when you are having a bad day.

I have found that an average, hard-working guy is only going to be able to restrict his caloric intake for about one hundred days per year. So let's say that during those hundred days he reduces his caloric intake by five hundred calories per day below what is needed to maintain his current weight. That would equal fifty thousand calories, which translates into a loss of about fourteen pounds (1 pound = 3,500 calories). Now let's also assume this person has 165 neutral days with his caloric intake equaling energy expenditure. During these days his weight would stay the same. That leaves one hundred days that the person would overeat to one degree or another. The ability to control his overeating on those bad dieting days is going to make or break the entire year. If this person overate by five hundred calories per day, it would nullify the weight loss during his good days. For weight loss to occur, the person would need to increase the number of neutral days and play defense on those bad days. It is not realistic to think that a person would be able restrict calories for more than a hundred days a year. A normal person with a real life is only going to be able to withstand a limited amount of days of restricting calories. Therefore, your good dieting days need to pay off. Playing defense and controlling the amount of overeating is the key. It is imperative that you don't give it all back by not playing defense. That would be like a football team orchestrating a fourteen-play scoring drive only to give it right back by allowing a touchdown on the following kickoff.

The idea is to gain back no more than 25 percent of the weight that was lost. You can say that this is a four-step-forward, one-step-back approach. Keep in mind that after three dieting cycles you would be nine steps forward. Let's look at a hypothetical example for a guy who happens to be twenty-five pounds overweight. During his first dieting cycle let's say that he loses fifteen pounds, and then during his off-season he regains four pounds. During his second dieting cycle he loses ten pounds, but this time he regains three pounds. By the third dieting cycle, he really starts to get the hang of it and proceeds to lose nine more pounds but only gains two of them back. That would be a twenty-five-pound net loss for the year. Not only is he at his ideal body weight, but he will also be healthier. Now armed with a solid diet plan, his weight will range only a few manageable pounds from his ideal weight for the rest of his life.

That, my fellow dieters, is the game plan. I am absolutely positive that most sports-minded guys can follow this plan successfully. The only thing that I am worried about is that you will try to do too much too soon.

Chapter 2: Keeping Score

The fundamental concept of keeping score will have a profound impact on your diet. In fact, keeping score is the single most important concept of this diet because it provides the accountability and the feedback that are crucial for dietary success. Quite simply, keeping score lets you know if you are winning or losing.

The concept of keeping score is in contrast to the idea of moderation. Many dieters try to lose weight by eating moderately. In other words, they watch what they eat hoping that they are doing enough to lose their excess fat. But why hope when you can know for sure? If you are not keeping score, it becomes difficult to know if you are winning or losing. On the other hand, keeping score tells you everything that you need to know. (I will explain how to keep score shortly.)

STATISTICS

In sports, more information is needed in addition to whether a team or individual has won or lost. It is really the statistics that account for the full understanding of the game. It is hard to imagine playing or watching sports without statistics. We are inundated with more statistics during a game than imaginable. During a game, we are accustomed to the announcer telling us the batting average of the second-string shortstop against left-handed pitchers with less than two outs and runners in scoring position. But the statistics regarding the food that goes into our mouths is another story. You can't go days, weeks, months, or years without you knowing the quality of food that is going down your throat. It is time to keep the statistics of your own diet. My point is this: it is difficult to improve your diet without knowing its details. Information about your current diet is vital. How would you like to rank a baseball player without knowing his batting average or a golfer without knowing his handicap? What would you say if a basketball player that you were coaching came up to you and said he wanted to average twenty points and eight rebounds a game for the next season — but when you asked him how many points he averaged during the last season, he would tell you that he doesn't know? And then when asked how many rebounds he grabbed, he would respond by asking, "What's a rebound?" Well, that scenario isn't much different from what is going on in the game of dieting. People are trying to lose weight and improve their diets without knowing the amount of calories or nutrients that they should be eating. You need to look at the statistics of your diet like the back of a baseball card. Instead of batting average, RBIs, and home runs, you will need to be monitoring things like calories, grams of protein, carbohydrates, fiber, and fats. Sure, it will take some work. But what of value doesn't? It's simply not right for someone to know everything about sports and nothing about the things he is putting into his mouth.

FOOD RANKINGS

The food rankings are designed to help you keep score of your diet and provide the necessary "statistics" of your meals. The food rankings are a listing of hundreds of food choices (e.g., meals, snacks, side orders, desserts, fruits) that have been rated as Gold, Silver, Bronze, or Zero-Value foods. You will find the food rankings in the back of the book (appendix E). The grouping of foods into four different categories gives you the opportunity to improve your diet choices one level at a time.

They also allow for the opportunity to learn about the nutrient content of the foods that you eat every day. The objective of the food rankings is for you to have a one-page snapshot view of forty-six different food groupings. By looking at the columns of various nutrients within a particular food group, you will be able to compare the differences between the Gold and lesser-ranked foods. This will give you a great idea of what to look for when choosing your meals. The objective of the food rankings is not to list every food that is available. The rankings are teaching tools, not menus. (Instructions on how to use the Internet to find the nutritional content of any food in the world will be discussed in the chapter titled Play Ball!)

The food rankings take the guesswork out of picking the proper foods to eat. They answer the number-one question that I have heard over the years: "So, what can I eat?" It's a great question. The Diet and Health Knowledge Survey of the United States Department of Agriculture (USDA) found that 80 percent of adults agreed with the statement that choosing a healthy diet is just a matter of knowing what foods are good or bad to eat.

The rankings of Gold, Silver, Bronze, or Zero-Value foods are determined by the effect these foods have on your total nutritional intake for the day. In other words, we want to know whether the selected food increases or decreases the likelihood that the dieter will stay within his recommended guidelines for the day. The better foods are ranked as Gold, followed by slightly lesser foods that are ranked as Silver. The next ranking is Bronze, which consists of foods that are inferior to both the Gold and Silver rankings, for one or more reasons. The final ranking is the Zero-Value foods, which, I'm sure you have guessed, have zero value and should only be eaten occasionally, if at all.

Keep in mind that these rankings are based mostly on common sense. Please don't blow a gasket if a food is placed in a category that you don't agree with. They are general guidelines designed to help simplify your food choices, not to add to the confusion. Your diet will be judged on whether it stays within the dietary guidelines as a whole, not on any one particular food.

Also keep in mind that in a capitalistic society, everyone has the right to make money producing delicious foods that are full of saturated fat, trans fat, and salt. The overconsumption of bad foods by the public is not the manufacturers' problem. You can't expect them to lose any sleep if these foods are making you unhealthy, fat, or prematurely dead. Their job is to make money; your job is to know exactly what is going into your mouth.

THE SCORECARD

Diet for the Sports-Minded Male will use two methods to keep score. The first method is the scorecard. During training camp, you will be asked to keep score of your new diet. To accomplish this, the foods that you select from the food rankings will be recorded onto your scorecard. A sample scorecard can be found in appendix B. The scorecard is designed to give you a clear picture of how your diet stacks up against the *Dietary Guidelines for Americans* for twelve key categories. It is a relatively easy way to get to a comprehensive understanding of your diet and learn a lot about foods in the process. I realize that there are computer programs and Web sites that can monitor your meals, but you will learn and remember so much more when you do it by hand.

The completion of a scorecard is rather simple. Many of the foods that you normally consume can be found in the food rankings, complete with all the nutritional information. All you need to do is record the information from the food rankings onto your scorecard. However, if a food is not found in the food rankings, you will have to obtain its information from the Nutrition Facts food label that is listed on the packages of most foods. After totaling the nutrients from all the foods consumed that day, you can easily determine if your diet is within the recommended dietary guidelines for the twelve nutritional categories that we will be monitoring. (Information regarding the *Dietary Guidelines* and the Nutrition Facts label will be provided shortly.)

The purpose of this book is not to blindly follow a diet, but rather to improve and learn about the foods that you eat on a regular basis. The scorecard is designed to tell you exactly where your diet stands. Your diet will either fall within the dietary guidelines or it won't. This makes it possible to deal with facts instead of assumptions. For example, the USDA's Diet and Health Knowledge Survey found that 58 percent of adults who assumed their caloric intake was about right were actually overeating. Similar realizations are often found in the world of sports. If you ever had your golf swing videotaped, you probably know what I mean. Most golfers are quite surprised by the fact that their swing isn't as picturesque as they imagined. Calculating the score of your diet may also provide some surprises.

THE SCALE

The second method of keeping score is the scale. There will be two weigh-ins each week, on the same days and at the same times. Twice per week seems to be the optimal number of times for weighing. More than twice a week is not necessary, while only once a week limits the feedback that is critical for timely alterations.

You may have heard that weighing yourself is not a good idea. Some believe that weight isn't important and shouldn't be stressed. Obviously, I disagree. Keep in mind that 75 percent of successful dieters who were able to lose thirty pounds or more and keep it off were in the habit of weighing themselves at least once a week. This statistic comes from the National Weight Control Registry and was developed to identify and investigate the characteristics of individuals who have succeeded at long-term weight loss. [2]

Weighing yourself is not supposed to be a traumatic experience. You are just supposed to hop on the scale and let it tell you how much you weigh. There is nothing to get bent out of shape about. Your weight *is* what it *is*. The numbers on the scale won't tell you if the weight lost or gained was from fat, water, or muscle. But if you are following the proper diet, you can rest assured that the weight lost will be from fat and the weight gained will be from muscle.

2. The National Weight Control Registry. 25 January, 2010
<http://www.nwcr.ws/>

Chapter 3:
Object of the Game

The object of this diet is to improve your food choices, one step at a time, until they adhere to the *Dietary Guidelines for Americans*.[3] These dietary guidelines will be the basis for the recommendations made in this book. Therefore, I feel that it's important to review how these guidelines and recommendations are made. The *Dietary Guidelines* are formulated, and revised every five years, by the joint effort of the U.S. Department of Agriculture (USDA) and the U.S. Department of Health and Human Services (HHS). Also assisting in the making of the guidelines is an external Dietary Guidelines Advisory Committee (DGAC) appointed by the USDA and the HHS to analyze all new pertinent scientific research. Since the year 2000, a significant amount of the recommendations made were based on the Dietary Reference Intake (DRI) reports. Briefly, the DRI is a combination of many reference values including the Recommended Dietary Allowance (RDA), Estimated Average Requirement (EAR), Adequate Intake (AI), Tolerable Upper Intake Level (UL), and the Acceptable Macronutrient Distribution Range (AMDR). Table 3-1 includes an explanation for these reference values. The main point is that millions of our tax dollars go into finding the best dietary recommendation for all Americans. The top nutritional experts and scientists are devoted to making America as healthy as it can be. That doesn't mean that these scientists agree on everything, but they certainly have developed

---

3. *Dietary Guidelines for Americans,*. 2005. Department of Health and Human Services. 24 January, 2010
<http://www.health.gov/dietaryguidelines/dga2005/document/default.htm>

the most comprehensive and scientifically based nutritional recommendations on Earth.

Hopefully, these recommendations will alleviate much of the confusion and controversy that surrounds the topic of nutrition. I believe that much of the confusion and controversy stems from diet books basing their recommendations on a limited amount of scientific research. Sure, there may be a few research articles supporting the plausibility of their claims, but all too often the research refuting those claims is omitted. You really need to look at the entire picture in a way that is fair and balanced. That's why it becomes imperative to review all the research and not just the few studies that happen to promote one side of a story.

I understand that it's nearly impossible to read every research article that is published. I also understand that hardly anyone would want to. But why not listen to the people who have? The *Dietary Guidelines* were formulated after analyzing *all* of the scientific research. The top scientists and nutritional experts examine all the facts and not just the convenient few that happen to advance one particular point of view. It's their job to develop the best possible recommendations for all Americans. The recommendations of this book are based on the *Dietary Guidelines for Americans* that were painstakingly developed by the leading nutritional agencies of the United States.

Table 3-1

Recommended Dietary Allowance (RDA) — the average daily nutrient level sufficient to meet the requirements of 98 percent of healthy individuals of a particular gender and age.

Adequate Intake (AI) — the average required daily nutrient level based on observed or experimentally determined approximations of intakes by a group of apparently healthy people. Used when RDA cannot be determined.

Tolerable Upper Intake Level (UL) — the highest average daily nutrient intake that is likely to pose no risk of adverse health effects to almost all individuals.

Estimated Average Requirement (EAR) — the average daily nutrient intake level estimated to meet the requirement of half the individuals of a particular gender and age.

Acceptable Macronutrient Distribution Range (AMDR) — is the range of a particular energy source that is associated with a reduced risk of chronic disease while providing intakes of essential nutrients. If an individual consumes in excess of the AMDR, there is a potential of increasing the risk of disease and/or insufficient intakes of other essential nutrients.

I have narrowed down their recommendations to twelve nutritional categories that we will monitor with the use of the scorecards. The idea is to monitor enough information to properly analyze your diet, while not making it so tedious that you won't do it.

The 12 Scorecard Nutritional Categories

Twelve separate nutritional categories, monitored during the first four weeks of training camp, will give you an excellent indication of the worthiness of your diet. This nutritional information will then be recorded onto your scorecards. The scorecards are designed to tell you the particulars of your diet and point out where you can make improvements. This system takes all the confusion out of dieting. Your diet will either fall into the recommended guidelines or it won't. There is nothing confusing about that. The goal is to have all twelve categories fall within the recommended dietary guidelines set by the USDA.

Let's review the twelve nutritional categories that we will be monitoring:

Calories (energy needs):

Many of the recommendations for the nutritional categories fall within a specific range. This is not the case with calories. Calorie requirements need to be more precise because excess amounts are stored as fat. The exact number of calories needed by an individual depends on many variables. Age, gender, height, and weight all influence the number of calories needed. The activity level of a person is another important consideration. Energy (calories) needed for a person who exercises strenuously will be drastically different from a couch potato of equal stature. Because of these many variables, you will be using a formula to calculate your caloric needs. These calculations will be done during the first days of training camp. This formula, called the Harris-Benedict Formula, takes into account a person's gender, height, weight, age, and activity level. The body composition of an individual will also have a great impact on caloric needs. Keep in mind that a pound of muscle takes roughly forty calories per day to maintain while a pound of fat takes only two. This formula does not account for the body composition of the dieter but nevertheless will provide us with enough information to plan a successful diet program.

Overall, calories are probably the most talked about, but neglected, aspect of dieting. Each person needs to know exactly how many calories they require to maintain, lose, or gain weight. This knowledge cannot be neglected.

Carbohydrates:
Recommended Range: 45–65 Percent

Carbohydrates have gotten a bad name over the past fifteen years. This bad reputation has come from the overconsumption of inferior carbohydrates, such as, snack foods, soda, pastries, processed grains, processed pastas, and a deluge of added sugars. These inferior carbohydrates should never be confused with "good" carbohydrates like fruits, vegetables, and whole grains. These superior carbohydrates have been the main source of energy for human beings since the beginning of time. Mankind still needs carbohydrates. Athletes depend on carbohydrates. Your body demands carbohydrates. The exact amount has been determined to be between 45 and 65 percent of your caloric intake.

If carbohydrates have been an essential part of humans' diet for millennia, and all athletes need them, then why, you may ask, have low-carbohydrate diets become popular? The popularity of low-carbohydrate diets is undoubtedly due to the promise of rapid weight loss. When carbohydrates are lacking, the body often goes into ketosis, which requires that the body break down its reserves of fat (a good thing) and muscle (not a good thing) in order to survive. Ketosis is a wonderful bodily function that is critical for survival, but it is not a way of life. Those that lose weight on low-carbohydrate diets eventually have to reenter the real world. When they do, they often regain the weight that they had lost at an alarming rate. This is not a scare tactic on my part or an attempt to stop anyone from trying these types of diets. No one can stop you from trying them; their allure is simply too great. I've tried them too. After all, who doesn't want to eat like a pig and still lose weight? But sooner or later we all have to learn to eat a healthy balanced diet. Also note that 99 percent of dieters who were able to lose thirty pounds or more and keep it off were *not* eating low-carbohydrate diets. These statistics were compiled by the National Weight Control Registry (http://www.nwcr.ws) that I referenced in the previous chapter.

Protein:
Recommended Range: 10–15 Percent

Protein has gotten its share of attention in the media, and rightfully so. It is indeed an important macronutrient that is necessary for growth and repair. Proteins also function as enzymes, hormones, and transport carriers. They are the major structural component of all cells and much more. But that doesn't mean that you should sit down and have nine steaks. The problem in America is not an insufficient protein intake; statistics show that the average intake for adults is more than the recommended amount. The problem is eating too much of the saturated fat and cholesterol that many sources of protein contain. Think about it. How many people do you know who have protein deficiencies? And how many people do you know are overweight? The main problem, for most people, is not an insufficient protein intake. Again, the problem for most of us is eating too much fat, saturated fat, and cholesterol with our protein.

For different individuals, the amount of protein needed can vary drastically. For the general population the recommended intake is 0.36 grams per pound of body weight (0.8g/kg). For those that work out intensely, the amount increases to 0.64 grams per pound of body weight (1.4g/kg) for endurance sports and 0.82 grams per pound of body weight (1.8g/kg) for resistance training.[4] These protein amounts can usually be reached by having 10 to 15 percent of your diet consisting of protein. In theory, the extra protein needed for training will be attained by the consumption of the additional calories needed

---

4. American Dietetic Association. Position of the American Dietetic Association, Dietitians of Canada and the American College of Sports Medicine. 25 January, 2010
<http://www.eatright.org/About/Content.aspx?id=8365> (PDF version, p.510)

for training. This is true in most cases, but not all. This will be explained in more detail a bit later.

Total Fat:
Recommended Range: 20–35 percent

A fear of fat has permeated the American conscience. This shouldn't be the case. Similar to carbohydrates, fat has gotten a bad reputation. Like carbohydrates, the bad reputation has come from the overconsumption of inferior fats, such as saturated and trans fats. This has resulted in people shying away from foods containing superior fats, such as avocados, nuts, peanut butter, and olive oil.

Fats are needed to supply energy for the body, protect internal organs, support the structure of cell membranes, and are essential for the absorption of fat-soluble vitamins. Of equal importance, fat provides taste and satiety to the diet. At the end of the day, you will be more likely to not exceed the right number of calories if your meals contain the proper amount of fat, since they will be tasty and satisfying.

It is certainly possible to be vibrantly healthy on a diet where 10 to 20 percent of calories come from fat. However, this is highly unlikely for a non-vegetarian male. For most of us, consuming less than 20 percent of calories from fat often leads to the overconsumption of inferior carbohydrates, a lack of taste, and a decreased capacity to feel full. The overconsumption of inferior carbohydrates can contribute to an increase in triglyceride levels that are associated with an increased risk of cardiovascular disease. This is especially ironic being that most people cut back on fat specifically to avoid heart trouble. On the other hand, fat consumption needs to be kept in check. Keeping fat between 20 and 35 percent can be challenging, especially when attempting to eat the recommended amount of calories. Fat calories can add up quite quickly due to the fact that a gram of fat equals nine calories, as compared to a gram of protein or carbohydrates, which equals four calories.

Saturated Fat:
Recommended Range: less than 10 percent of total calories

Let's start by calculating how much saturated fat we are talking about for an average guy that requires twenty-five hundred calories a day. Being that there are nine calories per gram of fat, the total number of grams recommended for this person would be twenty-eight grams of saturated fat or less (2,500 kcal x 10% = 250 kcal. ÷ 9 kcal/g = 28 g). To put this in perspective, consider that a Burger King biscuit with sausage, egg, and cheese has fourteen grams of saturated fat. Couple that wonderful breakfast (I'm being facetious) with a double cheeseburger for lunch, and voila, your total saturated fat intake is now maxed out for the day. Keep in mind that we have not added the saturated fat content for the french fries, cookies, milk shakes, or dinner and dessert. Major sources of saturated fat include cheese, beef, whole milk, oils, ice cream, cakes, cookies, and butter.

Cholesterol:
Recommended Range: less than 300mg per day

I'm sure you have seen the TV commercial explaining that there are two sources of cholesterol; your diet and the cholesterol produced by your liver. The commercial implies that the genes that you inherited from your family may have as much to do with your cholesterol levels as your diet. But let's not kid ourselves; our cholesterol levels have more to do with Ronald McDonald, Colonel Sanders, and Carl's Jr. than your genes.

Too much cholesterol in the blood can increase the risk of cardiovascular disease (CVD). Therefore, it is important that we limit the amounts of dietary cholesterol to 300mg per day. Cholesterol is a waxy substance needed to insulate nerves, make cell membranes and produce certain hormones. The main food sources are liver (370mg/3.5oz), whole eggs (250mg), meats (85mg/3.5oz), and milk products. Fruits and vegetables have zero cholesterol. Only animals can produce cholesterol.

Trans Fat:
Recommended Range: as low as possible (< 1 percent of total calories)

You'll be hearing a lot about trans fat in the years to come. The USDA suggests that you keep the intake of trans fats as low as possible. That's a nice way of saying, "this stuff is bad news." One by one, food manufacturers are taking all trans fat out of their products. Processed foods and oils provide roughly 80 percent of all trans fat, while 20 percent is derived naturally from animals. Common items that contain trans fat include margarine, fried potatoes, cakes, cookies, crackers, and pies. So start reading those food labels and keep this stuff to a minimum. Trans fat is now required to be listed on the Nutrition Facts label.

Keep in mind that companies can list the trans fat content as zero if the product contains less than one-half of a gram. Companies have been known to decrease the serving size in order to claim that their product doesn't contain trans fat, when it actually contains slightly less than a half a gram per serving. In many cases the person would unknowingly be eating approximately 0.4 grams of trans fat per serving. It's a good idea to check if the word "hydrogenated" is included in the ingredients. If it is, then the product has trans fat.

Fiber:
Recommended Range: 14 grams per 1,000 calories (35 grams is a nice, round number to keep in your head)

Don't start smirking when I mention fiber. I am not just talking about Granny's prune juice. This stuff is important. In fact, the quality of your diet depends crucially on its amount of fiber. The quantity of fiber you ingest certainly gives you a good indication of how many plant-based foods (fruits, vegetables, beans, whole grains, and oats) you are eating. Fiber is the part of the plant that is indigestible. Animal products, like meat, fish, chicken, and eggs, do not contain fiber. Quite often, plant-based foods are processed, removing much of the fiber. Therefore, to get a sufficient amount of fiber, you need to eat unprocessed plant-based foods, such as: whole wheat breads, cereals, and pasta; fruits; beans, and vegetables. In other words, if you are getting plenty of fiber (from food sources), chances are real good that your diet is healthy. Foods that contain fiber often have other valuable nutrients. Presently, the average amount of fiber consumed by Americans is less than half of the recommended amount.

Fiber has the capacity to slow digestion, making you feel fuller longer. Fiber can also lower cholesterol levels if combined with a healthy diet. Fibrous foods like oats, bran, beans, lentils, peas, apples, pears, strawberries, nuts, and seeds provide plenty of fiber and act like a sponge, absorbing cholesterol. Foods like whole grains, barley, brown rice, celery, tomatoes, beets, carrots, cabbage, cauliflower, and whole grain breakfast cereals improve digestion and prevent constipation. So, it may not sound very manly, but we are going to be paying close attention to our fiber.

Sugars:
Recommended Range: less than 25 percent of total calories

Sugars for this category are classified as monosaccharides or disaccharides. Monosaccharides and disaccharides are very small units of carbohydrate molecules often called simple sugars. Examples of foods that contain simple sugars are fruit and candy. This category does not include the larger molecules of carbohydrates called polysaccharides or complex carbohydrates. Examples of foods that contain complex carbohydrates (starch) are bread, pasta, rice, and cereals.

The problem with this classification is that it doesn't differentiate between the naturally occurring simple sugars found in an apple, for example, and sugars that are added to products like candy, cake, soda, and cookies. Also included in the list of added sugars are products with names like dextrose, sucrose, high fructose corn syrup, and maltose, to name a few. These are the types of sugars that should be limited to no more than 25 percent of your total calories. I happen to think that 25 percent is way too much, but we'll let that go for now.

Because of the discrepancy between naturally occurring simple sugars and added sugars, it is difficult to determine the optimal amount of sugars. However, common sense will tell you that the added sugars in soda and candy are the ones that should be limited.

Sodium:
Recommended Range: less than 2,300mg (about 1 teaspoon of salt)

Most of our sodium intake comes from the consumption of salt, which is a combination of sodium and chloride. Nearly all

Americans consume too much salt. This is problematic because, on average, the more salt a person consumes, the more likely he is of having high blood pressure. Keeping blood pressure in the normal range reduces the risk of heart and kidney disease. Now here's the catch. The majority of the salt that we consume does not come from the salt shaker. Adding salt to your food accounts for only 6 percent of salt intake. The overwhelming majority (77 percent) comes from processed foods. Many of the processed foods (e.g., potato chips, canned soups, fast food, frozen pizza, bread) have plenty of salt added during production. Therefore, the monitoring of salt intake becomes an excellent way to keep tabs of the amount of processed foods that you are eating. This category is similar to that of fiber; both give you a good indication of the caliber of your diet. Diets that are high in fiber and low in salt usually contain many healthy selections such as fruits, vegetables, beans, and whole grains while being limited in fast foods, canned foods, and processed foods.

Fruit and Vegetable Servings: Recommended Range: Fruits — between 2–4 servings; Vegetables — between 3–5 servings

I have added the categories of fruits and vegetables to the standard categories that are listed on the Nutrition Facts food label. Therefore, your scorecard will monitor the nutrients on the Nutrition Facts food label, plus two additional columns to denote how many servings of fruits and vegetables you are eating. I have done this in order to simplify matters. I'm sure that no one wants to monitor every vitamin, mineral, and antioxidant that is found in foods. In my estimation, it will be highly likely that you will be getting all your required vitamins, minerals, and antioxidants if you adhere to the recommended dietary guidelines. For example, if you are consuming the proper amount of calories and eating the proper amount of fruits and vegetables, then you will be automatically eating less processed foods and sodium, and more fiber, vitamins, minerals, and antioxidants. As an added bonus, you will also be eating more phytonutrients that are often found in fruits and vegetables. Phytonutrients, sometimes called phytochemicals, provide added health benefits above the nutrient value of the food. These phytochemicals have weird names that you may have heard on commercials, such as; carotenoids, flavonoids, lignans, and lycopene. Taking vitamin and mineral supplements is a good idea, but they don't compare with the nutritional value of fruits and vegetables.

It really isn't that difficult to consume the recommended amount of fruits and vegetables. Consider that one apple, pear, or small banana is one serving of fruit and that one ear of corn or a medium baked potato equals one serving of vegetables. Another option is to use frozen fruit to make smoothies. Did you know that one cup of frozen mango counts as two servings of fruit? If you add another cup of frozen banana or berries, you will have more than three fruit servings for the day.

The USDA recommends an exact number of fruit and vegetable servings for each individual depending on various factors. I personally don't get too hung-up about the exact number of servings. The point is to eat more fruits and vegetables. I suggest that you eat at least two servings of fruit and three servings of vegetables every day. Once you have reached that goal, try to eat as many as four servings of fruit and five servings of vegetables per day, as often as you can. It may take some work to get into the habit of having fruits and vegetables on a regular basis, but it is worth it.

Chapter 4:
Making Changes

The most difficult aspect of this diet plan is going to be choosing the appropriate changes that you will be making. No one else can possibly guess what changes you are ready to make or at what pace. The most important factor is for you to determine an appropriate change and then keeping track of whether you are executing the change or not. Accomplishing your goals is a great source of continued motivation. Competence breeds confidence and confidence is contagious.[5] The more goals that you accomplish, the more confidence you will gain. The key is to pick a challenging enough goal that will give you a sense of accomplishment. You will not feel a sense of accomplishment when the goal chosen is too easy. Conversely, you should not set yourself up for failure by choosing a goal that creates a sense of drudgery.

Here are a few tips to help you pick the appropriate changes:

TIP #1—Be patient. Generally speaking, sports-minded males aren't the most patient creatures on Earth. When starting a new venture, they often attempt to do too much, too soon. For example, the first day back in the weight room is usually followed by three days of not being able to move without something hurting. Guys can hear the story about the tortoise

---

5. I believe this term was coined by Dan Millman, author of *Way of the Peaceful Warrior* and many other great books.

and the hare until they are blue in the face and never be convinced that the turtle will win. But that's not going to stop me from reminding you again that slow and steady wins the race.

A marathon coach once said that you do not run twenty-six miles, rather you run one mile twenty-six times. I believe that his practical approach applies to dieting as well. In other words, you don't lose twenty-six pounds; you patiently lose one pound twenty-six times.

TIP #2 — Use the food rankings (appendix E). One of the best ways to make changes is to select food choices from the Gold and Silver sections of the food rankings. Simply browse the food rankings and pick foods that you like which have a higher ranking than the foods you are currently eating.

TIP #3 — Make a habit of reading food labels. The more that you know about the nutrients that are in foods, the better able you will be at choosing properly. Food manufacturers are required to display the content of their food on the Nutrition Facts label. This policy was instituted to help educate the American public and make an impact on the rising rate of obesity. Unfortunately that didn't happen. In fact, the obesity rate kept rising (it has currently leveled off). The fact is that most people don't read the label. The slogan "read it before you eat it" seems to have been replaced with "those that need it don't read it."

Knowing the nutritional content of each individual food that you are eating is beneficial. But knowing the nutritional content of your entire day is priceless. That is the purpose of the scorecard. Everything that you eat during the day will be recorded onto the scorecard so that you can judge your entire day. Your scorecard will have your goals for the day listed on the bottom. All you have to do is compare them with what you actually ate. It's that easy, especially after you have done it a few times.

TIP #4 — Familiarize yourself with the Zero-Value foods of the food rankings. Check out the astonishing nutritional content of some of these foods. Ask yourself, "Do I still want to eat these inferior foods after knowing what's in them?"

TIP #5 — Rank the foods that you are currently eating according to your attachment to them. You need to make an honest evaluation to distinguish between inferior foods that you love and have no intention of eliminating and the inferior foods that you can do without. My suggestion is to first eliminate the foods that lack an emotional attachment. For example, if you eat ice cream often and absolutely can't live without it, then by all means continue. Limit the amount, but continue. But if you can do without it, then discontinue having it. Or you may want to consider switching to low-fat ice cream, frozen low-fat yogurt, or low-cal fruit or fudge pops.

TIP #6 — Keep your focus on the foods that you want and not on the foods that you are trying to limit or avoid. Try not to dwell or obsess on the foods that you will be giving up. A racecar driver doesn't go around the track thinking about not hitting the wall. A golfer visualizes the ball landing on the fairway; he does not visualize it sailing into the woods. You will attract what you think about, whether it is good for you or not. That's why trying not to eat something doesn't work. Focus on the foods that you enjoy that are part of your new and improved diet. For example, you should say to yourself, "I can't wait to have oatmeal when I wake up; it is so good" and not, "I sure miss my doughnuts."

TIP #7 — Try meal replacement drinks. With all this talk about food choices you may find it helpful to consider meal replacement drinks. They can be very helpful due to their convenience and nutritional value. Active guys often find it difficult to prepare four to six meals or snacks per day. Without relying on replacement drinks, many find it difficult to consume the needed amount of protein without having excessive amounts of saturated fat and cholesterol. Meal replacement drinks can be a big help.

TIP #8 — Don't try to be perfect. No matter how hard you try, mistakes will happen. Sports are often a succession of good plays, great shots, big hits, and fantastic catches intertwined with broken plays, bad shots, strikeouts, and dropped balls. And diets are often a succession of good food choices followed by some bad choices. In other words, mistakes are part of the game. Athletes are accustomed to making mistakes and then forgetting about them quickly. The next play is coming fast and the past needs to be forgotten in a hurry. In sports, this is called having a short memory. Having a short memory is helpful in the game of dieting. Mistakes are part of the game. Approaching a diet without this realization can be devastating.

TIP #9 — Try fruit smoothies. Fruit smoothies can be had for breakfast, lunch, or snacks. Just like the meal replacement drinks, they add to your food choices and are also convenient. Unlike fresh fruit, frozen fruits rarely go bad and are always available. And they are a great way to get the required amount of fruit servings. Fruit is considered a good source of carbohydrates that is full of vitamins, minerals, and fiber. The scorecard will be tracking your fruit consumption. Smoothies are a great way to reach your goal. Remember to add a protein source to your smoothie (e.g., low-fat yogurt or protein powder) to create a balanced meal. You can also add one hundred calories of extra-firm tofu for an additional ten grams of protein. I know it sounds gross, but you should try it. Trust me on this one.

TIP #10 — Have designated times for meals and snacks. In other words, only eat during your designated times. This is great way to stop the habit of grazing. We are not cows. This is also a helpful way to give your diet some structure. For example, do not eat a single piece of food for three hours following lunch. You can then have a snack and then continue not to eat anything for the two to three hours before dinner. These "Do Not Eat Zones" can help give your diet some structure. With a little practice you will get better at planning the appropriate size meals and snacks that will keep you satisfied but not stuffed throughout the day.

TIP #11—Don't tell anybody that you are on a diet, because you are not. You are simply improving the way that you are eating. This is about you and your health. It is nobody else's business. Simply stick to your plan, methodically and quietly.

TIP #12—Ask yourself this simple question, "What would I be eating if I were already at my ideal weight?" Never forget that you already know more than you think. You know yourself better than anyone else. Don't sell yourself short. You may not know everything about nutrition (who does?), but you probably know more than enough to improve your health.

Chapter 5: Trick Plays

Sports teams always have a few trick plays under their sleeves. *Diet for the Sports-Minded Male* has a few of its own. No matter how fundamentally sound your game plan may be, it is always nice to be able to rely on a few trick plays.

   The Twenty-Minute Rule—I don't recall when I first heard about the twenty-minute rule, but it's a good one. This rule alone can make a dramatic impact on your health. The rule suggests that you wait twenty minutes before having a second helping of a meal or before having dessert. The idea is to fill your plate with an appropriate serving size. After the meal is consumed, you should allow twenty minutes to pass before eating anything else. If you are still hungry after the twenty minutes then feel free to have more. There will be times when you will be legitimately hungry after the twenty minutes, but I'm certain that the majority of the time you'll get the feeling of satisfaction and not have to eat anymore. The rationale is to give your stomach enough time to tell your brain that you are full. Most guys will always feel hungry when they are in the process of eating. You need to stop eating in order to tell if you are full. This may sound strange, but I think you'll find out that it is true. The process of eating is actually making you hungrier. Have you ever wondered why you can eat non-stop on Thanksgiving Day? It's when you stop eating that you can begin to feel full. Don't wait until you feel like you are going to explode before you stop. Your brain needs to tell you that you are full, not your stomach. Stomachs can hold way more than you need. Feeling full should be a mental thing, not a physical thing.

The 80 Percent Rule—This rule can be implemented once you are convinced that the twenty-minute rule is of value. Not only does it take about twenty minutes to realize that you are full, but often it will only take about 80 percent of the foods that you think. As the saying goes; our eyes are bigger than our stomachs. So try it out. Eat only 80 percent of what you would normally eat, then wait twenty minutes and see if you still feel like eating. You may be surprised. If you still feel hungry or deprived, then you can always eat some more.

The Munch and Crunch—This trick is great for guys who love to eat. Many of us, especially when ravenously hungry, have a tendency to eat with gusto. Some may say that we eat like animals. I happen to think that there is nothing wrong with enjoying a good meal. The problem is that there are many types of food that shouldn't be attacked when we are in a ravenous state. These foods are high in calories and too much damage can be done before you begin to feel satisfied. The foods that shouldn't be attacked are foods like pizza, cheese, bread baskets, chips and guacamole, nuts, fries, burgers, and a host of other foods. This rule suggests that you "munch and crunch" away on some safer foods until those animalistic tendencies have subsided. You may find it helpful to have a salad or soup before dinner. You may also "munch and crunch" on an apple or other fruit before dinner is served. Those one hundred calories provided by fruit may save you from overeating three hundred excess calories during dinner. Besides, you probably can use some fruit. Carrot or celery sticks are other good foods to munch on before a meal.

Lay Off the Diet Soda—It is advisable to lay off the diet soda and all other artificially sweetened foods. The suggestion to avoid these products is not only because of their chemical and caffeine content. The reason has more to do with the effect these products have on your taste buds. Diet soda is much sweeter than table sugar and fruits. Therefore, you will lose the desire for the naturally sweetened foods. Foods such as fruit will taste very bland to anyone accustomed to eating artificially sweetened foods. I am also concerned with the psychological need to have something in your mouth all day long. Do you really need to suck on an "adult baby bottle" disguised as a noncaloric beverage?

Three Big Meals versus Four to Six Small Meals—We have been hearing for years that eating smaller meals, more frequently, is beneficial for our health. The premise behind this pattern of eating is that your blood sugar level and hormone balance will remain optimal while not becoming overly hungry or irritable. Experts agree that this approach is a good idea for most people. The problem is that *most* people are not *all* people. Having three larger meals a day may be better for some. I say this because eating four to six smaller meals or snacks means that you will have to *stop* eating four to six times a day. For many, that is a problem. The potential is there to overeat four to six times a day rather than three. Also, with mini-meals, there is the possibility that you never feel quite satisfied and remain constantly anxious, anticipating the next feeding. Finally, much more planning and preparation is involved in trying to organize four to six meals. You may feel more satisfied eating three meals a day totaling twenty-five hundred calories, rather than overeating four to six meals totaling three thousand calories. The trick is to figure out which is right for you.

Crunch Time—Sports fans are well aware of crunch time. It's the time when the game is on the line and you expect your team to rise to the occasion. Careers are made or ruined according to how a player performs in the clutch. Taking the last shot in a basketball game or being at the plate with runners on second and third with two outs in the bottom of the ninth are scenarios that constitute crunch time for the athlete. Well, dieters have crunch times too.

Let's say you are out to eat and have finished a great meal. You are completely satisfied when the waiter asks if anyone would like dessert. That's crunch time for a dieter. What do you do? Crunch time could happen in your office. You are minding your own business, doing your job, and then all of a sudden you are offered a chocolate glazed donut. This is another example of crunch time. Know that they are coming and be prepared. Just silently say to yourself, "This is crunch time," then act the way you expect your sports teams to act. Don't you think it is a bit hypocritical to chastise your sports team for not performing under pressure when you melt at the sight of a donut?

Glycemic Index—You may have heard about something called the Glycemic Index (GI) and Glycemic Load (GL). They both measure the speed in which carbohydrate foods affect your blood glucose (sugar) levels. The GI deals with a set amount (50 grams) of individual carbohydrate foods while the GL measures the effect of an amount of a carbohydrate that are typically eaten as part of a meal. Glucose (sugar) entering the blood too quickly is not a good thing. Foods that break down and enter the bloodstream quickly are said to have a high glycemic index. The hormonal response to a rapid influx of sugar into the blood is increased levels of insulin, possibly producing a hypoglycemic state, or low blood sugar. In laymen terms, this translates to a sugar rush (buzz) followed by a crash, with symptoms like dizziness, tiredness, or irritability.

In the past, sugars were categorized as simple or complex carbohydrates. It was believed that simple sugars, like the ones in fruit and candy, entered the bloodstream faster than the ones in complex carbohydrates (e.g., baked potatoes). This theory has been proven false; many complex carbohydrates actually enter the bloodstream quite fast. Many books have theorized that avoiding foods with a high glycemic index (GI) will promote weight loss. Even though the overall evidence does not support these claims[6], it remains a good idea not to overindulge in high GI foods like fruit juice, soda, baked potatoes, white bread, white rice, and rice cakes. Limiting these foods as well as having high-GI foods as part of a balanced meal or snack will guard against the adverse effects that these foods can have on your blood sugar levels. For example, having one rice cake with a little bit of peanut butter will have less of a negative affect on your blood sugar level than having two rice cakes by themselves. In conclusion, I suggest that you don't become overly obsessed about the glycemic index. Just use a little common sense. For those that wish to learn more, you can go to *The Official Web site of the Glycemic Index and GI Database*. The Web site address is: http://www.glycemicindex.com/

Sit and Eat—Quite often our eating has nothing to do with true hunger. Many times we eat because we are excited, anger, worried, anxious, happy, or any number of other reasons. There is a trick to help you realize if you are eating for a reason other than the physiological need for nourishment. The trick is to pick a day that you eat all of your meals while seated and doing nothing else except eating: no watching TV, no reading the newspaper, and no text messaging. Just sit there and eat. If you would rather be doing something else, then do it. When you are truly hungry, you will stop and eat. If you try to do this a few times, you will start to realize that much of what you eat is for reasons other than true hunger. Vendors at ballparks will tell you that they do the best business during close games. Fans get excited and anxious and they comfort themselves with food. It's quite all right to eat like that, but at least be aware that you are not really hungry.

---

6. American Dietetic Association. Position of the American Dietetic Association: Weight Management. 24 January 2010 <http://www.eatright.org/About/Content.aspx?id=8382> (PDF version, p.334)

Chapter 6:
A Word about Exercise

Thank goodness that the sports-minded male knows a thing or two about exercise. Nevertheless, I would like to explain a few things about exercise as it relates to this diet. The main points I would like to make are listed below:

Point #1

You can't outrun dietary mistakes. Using exercise alone to lose weight is hopeless. I'll say it again; using exercise alone to lose weight is hopeless. It's not going to happen, unless you feel like running a marathon every week. Don't get me wrong; exercise is important, but it can only do so much. Both diet and exercise are needed for successful weight loss.

Point #2

Do not increase the intensity of your fitness program at the same time you are trying to improve your diet. Combining the two tasks is asking for trouble. Dieting and exercise should have an inverse relationship. When the focus for one is high, the intensity for the other should be low. You are not a professional boxer with a training staff and posse preparing for an upcoming fight. You have a real life and need real solutions. An appropriate challenge for a professional athlete is not appropriate for a sports-minded male with a real job.

I realize that this opposes everything that you have ever heard about getting back into shape. Typically, a dieter attempts to work out like a maniac in order to burn as many calories as possible. I am suggesting that this approach is a big-time mistake.

Point #3

Center your fitness program on the exercises that you like to do. People often want to know the best exercise. I answer that it is the exercise that they enjoy. As with diets, what good is designing a perfect diet if the person is not going to eat it on a regular basis? Well, the same goes for exercise. Doing the exercise that you like on a regular basis is going to be more advantageous than doing the so-called perfect exercise sporadically.

Point #4

Touch all the bases. You still need to combine what you like with what you need. We all need cardiovascular conditioning, muscular strength, and flexibility. All three facets of fitness need to be addressed. For example, if you like running, you are going to need to balance your running workouts with some strength training and flexibility. Focusing on your strength and flexibility is going to help you remain healthy enough to continue to do the exercises that you like. Those that enjoy weight training need to keep this in mind. Quite often, the cardiovascular conditioning is the Achilles' heel of the weight lifting enthusiast. The body's inability to deliver oxygen to the muscle (due to poor cardiovascular conditioning) can often be the reason for limited muscle growth. Flexibility training and working the muscle to its full range of motion is also beneficial for those weight training.

Point #5

Mix it up. You may find it difficult, if not impossible, to find the time to touch all the bases. A person may want to complete four cardiovascular workouts a week, weight train three times, and play golf or tennis on the weekends. This is not very practical for a busy person and something will have to give. My advice is to mix it up by changing your priorities throughout the year. Not all three facets of fitness can be the top priority at all times. For example, a runner may want to join a health club during the cold winter to work on his strength and flexibility. During this time he could maintain his running form by exercising on the treadmill. He could work on his leg strength by using traditional weights or using the treadmill for hill training. Likewise, someone who weight trains religiously may want to get outside during the warmer months to partake in mountain biking, jogging, rollerblading, or hiking. Mixing it up will help keep all facets of your fitness program fresh.

THE THREE FITNESS PHASES

We are now going to integrate these five points into the dieting cycles. The dieting cycles will be broken down into three fitness phases. Throughout the dieting cycles there will be an inverse relationship between dieting (focus on food) and exercise. During the times that you will be focusing on your diet you will not be adding to that burden by exercising like a madman. You will be exercising, but not at high intensity. Let's take a look at how this works.

PHASE ONE – TRAINING CAMP (WEEKS 1–8)

The goal of phase one is to exercise at a low-to-moderate intensity. This strategy increases the blood flow to the muscles, improves immune function, strengthens the heart, and prepares the body for more intense exercise down the road. During this phase, we are more concerned with increasing the number of times that you work out per week (frequency) and increasing the length of time of each workout (duration) than we are about increasing the intensity.

The low-to-moderate intensity is a challenging but comfortable effort that still enables you to have a conversation. In other words, comfortable enough to have a conversation, but challenging enough that you don't want to. This level is known as the upper limit of your aerobic range. Aerobic means "with oxygen", therefore you are working out at a pace that is challenging but still supplying sufficient oxygen to the muscles.

An extra bonus of this moderate intensity is that it burns the most fat. Note that I said the most fat rather than the highest percentage of fat. Guys normally don't fall for the trap suggesting that you work out at very low intensities in order to burn the highest percentage of fat. I don't care as much about the percentage, I care most about the total amount of fat and calories expended. After all, it's better to burn five hundred calories of which 50 percent is fat (250 kcal of fat), than two hundred calories of which 70 percent is fat (140 kcal of fat.)

That's your goal during phase one. You are preparing your body for the more demanding workouts to come while burning the maximum amount of fat. Plus, this allows the primary focus during training camp to be geared toward the improvement of your diet. When you are ready to focus on your fitness, you will be lighter and physiological prepared for the higher intensity workouts.

PHASE TWO—THE SEASON (weeks 9–12)

You are now prepared to enter phase two of your fitness program. Now is the time to push the envelope a bit. I call it entering the "uncomfortable zone," when you are exercising without being able to have a conversation without gasping. This is better known as anaerobic exercise, which means "without oxygen." This type of effort should be introduced slowly into your routine and only amount to a small percentage (10-15 percent) of the entire workout. If you are a walker, runner, or cyclist, this is the time to introduce a few hills or a few sprints into your routine.

PHASE THREE—THE OFF-SEASON (weeks 13-16)

During the off-season, your motivation toward dieting will probably start to wane—it's only natural. That makes it the perfect time to work out at top intensity. Now you can feel free to let it all hang out and to work out as long and hard as you would like.

You have diligently focused on improving your diet and losing weight. Now is time to switch your enthusiasm toward exercise. The extra calories that you may consume during the off-season will likely be offset by the additional calories that are needed to fuel your intense workouts. But don't expect that a few extra calories burned during exercise will compensate for a complete pig-out. It's not going to happen.

Most likely you will have to play a little defense during the off-season. Recall the advantages of playing defense from chapter one. A good thing to keep in mind during the off-season is the improbability of exercising away the excess calories that you consume. Let's do the math. An average-sized guy is going to burn about fifteen calories per minute jogging at a nine-minute-per-mile pace, equaling nine hundred calories for one hour. Weight training expends about ten calories per minute, which adds up to six hundred per hour. To put this into perspective, realize that this same person burns about 1.5 calories per minute sitting on the couch, which amounts to ninety calories an hour. Keep these numbers in mind before deciding to indulge in foods that you really don't need. The amount of calories that are in foods needs to be respected. Take the time to think of how hard it is to lose weight and how easy it is to gain it. Do you really want to neutralize an entire day of exercising by eating something you won't thoroughly enjoy? Check out the calories of what you are about to eat and decide for yourself. Is the buttered popcorn at the movies really worth an hour jog at a nine-minute-per-mile pace?

Chapter 7: Play Ball!

OK guys, you are finally ready to start the first sixteen-week dieting cycle. Ideally, a dieting cycle would begin in January, May, or September, but it really doesn't matter. What matters most is that you start. You can always adjust the length of your first few dieting cycles until they coincide with the dates that I have suggested. After gaining experience with this diet, you will eventually choose the starting dates and lengths of each dieting cycle to suit your personal preferences. Variations to the standard sixteen-week dieting cycle will be discussed at the end of the book.

As you may recall, the first eight weeks of a dieting cycle will be training camp, followed by a four-week season, and then the four-week off-season. The next dieting cycle begins immediately after the off-season of the previous dieting cycle. The idea behind *Diet for the Sports-Minded Male*, once again, is to make improvements to your diet in a step-by-step fashion and to increase the awareness of your food choices. Therefore, do not be alarmed that many of the recommendations for improving your diet seem easy to accomplish and that you feel that you could do more. Well, I know that you can do more. But the idea is not to prove how much you can withstand. The idea is to create a method that will get you into shape for the rest of your life.

The main objective of this first week is to select a more nutritious breakfast than you are currently eating. It will take the whole week to try a few new breakfast choices before settling on one that you like enough to eat on a regular basis. This is the week that will require the most patience. Remember the movie *The Karate Kid*. Well this is the "wax on, wax off" portion of your diet.

This method to get in shape is probably brand new for most of you. For starters, no one is going to be telling you what to eat as if you were ten years old. I'll say it one more time: This is going to be your diet, not mine. All the tools are here for you to improve your diet one step at a time at your own pace. Just keep in mind that there is no need to rush. You'll be eating every day for the rest of your life, so take your time.

To get a better idea of how this diet works, I have included examples of three typical sports-minded males. We learn so much in sports by watching others. That is what we hope to accomplish with the examples of our three "teammates." Included as part of the instructions for each week of the dieting cycle, I will use the examples for Fast-Food Freddy, Snack-Happy Steve, and Duck-Hook Harry. You will probably be faced with many similar problems to the ones they are facing. Seeing how they handle their challenges will give you some good ideas regarding how to handle yours. Allow me to introduce you to Freddy, Steve, and Harry.

Fast-Food Freddy

Freddy has been out of college for six years and is primarily concerned with his career. All of his competitive energy, which once was directed into sports, is now being funneled into his work. Freddy realizes that he is not twenty-two years old any longer and that his once excellent physique is getting more and more difficult to achieve. In top shape, Freddy weighed 175 pounds but is now tipping the scales at nearly 200 pounds. His nutritional knowledge is limited and he pretty much eats what he has always eaten, primarily because it tastes good. He has always been relatively healthy with no reason to change, until now. He is feeling sluggish and fat and can't stand it any longer. He lives alone and has a steady girlfriend that he sees occasionally during the week but mostly on weekends. He is not about to start cooking meals for himself and has no intention of eating anything like tofu, cottage cheese, yogurt, skim milk, or any other girlie foods.

Snack-Happy Steve

Steve is thirty-eight years old and happily married to Sally. They have two young boys, eleven and thirteen years of age. Sally is a typical soccer mom that makes sure that traditional sit-down dinners are prepared every night. She is fairly knowledgeable about nutrition and takes pride in feeding her family healthy meals. Steve is a salesman that works out of his home most of the time, traveling occasionally.

Steve played high school baseball but never got himself into great shape. In fact, his friends used to kid him about having "Pudgekins Disease" which is a terminal case of always looking pudgy no matter how hard you diet and exercise. He has currently pudged himself up to 240 pounds which is a tad much for his barely six foot frame.

Steve works without an assistant, spending much of his time making calls to his customers along with the necessary correspondence. His job is often stressful, leading him down the hall and into the well-stocked kitchen for snacks and treats that are supposed to be for the kids. His diet, in general, is not bad. His biggest problem is too many snacks, too much dessert, and too many second helpings.

Duck-Hook Harry

Harry is a recently divorced, fifty-two-year-old attorney who enjoys nothing more than a round of golf, followed by a round of drinks. The fact that Harry has not mastered the game of golf has not dampened his enthusiasm. He continues to enjoy every round of golf no matter how many drives he "duck hooks" into the trees. What he does not enjoy are the nagging pains that are becoming more persistent with each passing year. His lack of exercise, other than golf, and poor diet are starting to catch-up with good ole Harry. The extra ten pounds that he once carried without concern has now ballooned to thirty uncomfortable pounds. The extra weight coupled with the reoccurring aches and pains have finally gotten his attention. The motivation to improve his health is quite simple; he wants to continue to play the game he loves, without pain. Losing the belly will also have its advantages as he reenters the dating scene after twenty-four years of marriage. A better diet and some exercise is just what the doctor ordered.

Let us now begin our first eight-week training camp, one step at a time:

STEP #1

The first thing you have to do is figure out how many calories you require for one day. The calories needed are going to vary depending on your activity level. You will have different calorie needs depending on whether you are sedentary, lightly active, moderately active, or extremely active. This will be done by using the Harris-Benedict Formula. This formula takes into account your sex, age, height, weight, and activity level. The first part of the formula calculates your Basal Metabolic Rate (BMR). The BMR is the number of calories needed to maintain your current body weight if you stayed motionless in bed all day. Few people have this luxury, so the BMR then needs to be multiplied by the level of activity.

Keep in mind that this formula doesn't account for a person's body composition. In other words, it doesn't differentiate between a body that is 10 percent body fat versus a body of identical weight that is 30 percent body fat. Therefore, a person with more muscle will require more calories for a given day than a person with more fat (as I have already mentioned, a pound of muscle requires about forty calories a day to maintain, while a pound of fat needs only two). Therefore, the caloric needs that are calculated with this formula are estimates. Very good estimates, but estimates just the same.

There is also a USDA Web site that will do the calculations for you. But first let me explain how to do it using the Harris-Benedict Formula. Don't freak out, it's not as complicated as it looks:

The Harris Benedict Formula for Men:

BMR = 66 + (6.23 x Weight in pounds) + (12.7 x Height in inches) – (6.8 x Age in years)
Example: Let's calculate the BMR for Snack-Happy Steve who is 6'0" (72 inches), weighs 240 pounds, and is 38 years old.
BMR for Steve: 66 + (6.23 x 240lbs) + (12.7 x 72 inches) – (6.8 x 38 years old)

BMR = 66 + (1495.2) + (914.4) – (258.4)

BMR = 2475.6 – 258.4

BMR = 2,217 calories (kcal) per day

Now we need to add in the activity levels:
Sedentary = BMR x 1.2

Steve's daily caloric needs for a *sedentary* week would be:

BMR of 2,217 kcal. multiplied by 1.2 = **2,260 kcal.**
Light Activity = BMR x 1.375

A week with light activity (1-3 days of light exercise), daily caloric needs for Steve would be: BMR of 2,217 kcal. multiplied by 1.375 = **3,049 kcal.**

(Steve is going to use this activity level for his scorecards)
Moderate Activity = BMR x 1.55

A week of moderate activity (3-5 days per week), the daily caloric needs for Steve would be: BMR of 2,217 kcal. multiplied by 1.55 = **3,436 kcal**.

Very Active = BMR x 1.725

A week of being very active (hard exercise 6-7 times per week), Steve's daily caloric requirements would be: BMR of 2,217 kcal. multiplied by 1.725 = **3,824 kcal.**

Extra Active = BMR x 1.9

A week of extra activity (very hard exercise & physical job or exercising 2 times/day) Steve's daily caloric requirements would be: BMR of 2,217 kcal. multiplied by 1.9 = **4,212 kcal.**

(If a female wishes to use this diet, the equation is: BMR = 655 + (4.35 x weight in pounds) + (4.7 x height in inches) – (4.7 x age in years)).

Determining caloric needs using the USDA (Food and Nutrition Information Center) Web site:

1. Go to the homepage with the address: http://fnic.nal.usda.gov/.
2. On the left side of the page click on *Dietary Supplements*.
3. Then in the middle of the page (about half way down) click on *Macronutrients*.
4. Then scroll down under the heading of General Information and click on *Daily Nutrition Calculator (Macronutrients)*.
5. Simply fill in the requested information (height, weight, age, sex, activity level, etc.). Note: At this point of our program you will select that you wish to maintain your current weight.

Please note: the caloric needs calculated by this Web site will be slightly different from those determined by the Harris-Benedict Formula. If you happen to calculate both, simply use the lower amount. Keep in mind that both methods are estimates. At the end of the day, the scale is going to be the final judge as to your precise caloric needs. For example, if someone is gaining weight, it goes to reason that they are eating too many calories. At that point, it doesn't matter what these calculations are stating. The scale will be the final judge. These calculations are simply a good starting point.

Now is the time to start filling out your scorecards. This is also a good time to make some photocopies of the two scorecards we are going to use most often. The two scorecards can be found as appendix B and appendix C or downloaded from http://www.rayoflife.com. Appendix B is titled Scorecard—Meals and Snacks and appendix C is titled Scorecard—Totals for the Day. You will need two scorecards titled Scorecard—Totals for the Day and six scorecards titled Scorecard—Meals and Snacks.

The first thing you are going to do is record the calories needed for one day (calculated from the Harris-Benedict Formula or the Web site) and record that amount onto your scorecards. Then write down your activity level and the calorie goal. Keep in mind that the calorie amounts that we will use are for a person to maintain his body weight. We will be subtracting five hundred calories a day from these totals when the time comes (weeks 5-8 of training camp), but not now.

STEP #2

After calculating your caloric needs, you then need to find the amount of nutrients that are needed for each of the twelve nutrients that we will be monitoring. These amounts can be found in appendix A, titled Dietary Guidelines for Various Calorie Needs.

The amounts or ranges for each of the twelve nutritional categories, according to the calories that you need, will now be recorded onto a scorecard titled Scorecard — Totals for the Day, which can be found in appendix C. Record all twelve of your nutritional guidelines on the row near the bottom of the page, titled "Goal." These twelve categories are calculated to adhere to the *Dietary Guidelines for Americans*. The various calories needed for a day are listed in the left-hand column. The required range of nutrients follows each caloric amount that is required for the day. If your calorie needs fall between the amounts listed on appendix A, simply estimate your personal ranges for each category. When in doubt, choose the lower amount (except for fiber).

Special note: Notice that appendix A, Dietary Guidelines for Various Calorie Needs, has two columns for protein. One column is the recommended range and the other is the acceptable macronutrient distribution range. The acceptable range for protein is between 10 and 35 percent.[7] This range denotes the amount of protein that can be consumed without increasing the risk of disease or causing a deficiency of other essential nutrients. However, the recommended range of protein is between 10 and 15 percent. This is the typical amount of protein consumed by healthy individuals. I recommend that everyone begin the dieting cycle using the recommended range of 10 to15 percent.

The acceptable range for protein may be used for those exercising intensely. The calculation for the general public is 0.36

7. FNIC (Food and Nutrition Information Center) provides links to the DRI (Dietary Reference Intakes) Tables, developed by the Institute of Medicine's Food and Nutrition Board. 24 January, 2010
<http://www.iom.edu/Global/News%20Announcements/~/media/C5CD 2DD7840544979A549EC47E56A02B.ashx>

grams of protein per pound of body weight. For those who partake in endurance type exercise, the calculation would be 0.64 grams per pound of body weight. The protein requirements increase even more for those lifting weights intensely. The amount of protein needed for resistance type training goes up to 0.82 grams per pound of body weight. I would also add that these calculations should be made using your ideal body weight. The rationale being that the extra fat that you have doesn't require extra protein. For example, Snack-Happy Steve is 240 pounds. If he were to start a rigorous weight-training program during the off-season, he would want to consume 0.82 grams of protein per pound. If we used his current weight of 240 pounds, that would add-up to be 197 grams of protein. What I am recommending is that he uses his ideal weight of 190 pounds. That would calculate to be 156 grams of protein, which is more than enough to support his lean body mass minus the fat.

I mentioned early that the recommended range of 10 to 15 percent protein doesn't always provide the correct amount of protein for those exercising intensely. In the example above, Steve's protein needs were calculated to be 156 grams, which is 20 percent of the 3,049 calories he would need to maintain his weight. If he were to restrict his calories to 2,000 a day, the 156 grams of protein would be the equivalent of 31 percent. As you can see, the actual amount of protein remained constant while the percentage increased. In both cases, the amount of protein was higher than the recommended range of 10 to 15 percent. I suggest that everyone start the first dieting cycle with the goal of consuming between 10 and 15 percent of protein. Recall that this is not the time to work out intensely or to restrict calories.

STEP #3

Let's start by making improvements or changes to what you are currently eating for breakfast. The improvement that you make for breakfast should be applied for at least five days of the week. For example, you may elect to make a change to your new and improved breakfast Monday through Friday and continue with your old breakfast on the weekends. Some people benefit by indulging a bit on the weekends, while others would rather continue eating the healthier breakfast for the entire week. Depending on the type of person you are, you may choose either approach. These are the types of choices that only you can make. But the goal is to make your improvements for at least five days of the week. The changes that you make can range from switching from a donut to a bagel or switching from a sugary children's cereal to a healthier cereal with more whole grain and fiber. Another example of a typical change would be adding a glass of orange juice or using 2% milk instead of whole milk. I will use Fast-Food Freddy, Snack-Happy Steve, and Duck-Hook Harry as examples so that you can get a feel for how this is done.

During this first week, you are going to have to fight the tendency to want to change all your meals at once; that's not the method you want to use. This type of gradual approach is going to help in the future, making it much easier to re-start your diet after the off-season. You will no longer have to psych yourself up for days before starting a typical overly strict diet plan. Besides, this is training camp, which is a time to not only eat better, but also learn about the nutritional content of the food. The goal is not to turn your world up-side down, but rather to improve your diet with a steady, stealth-like transition. That is why you are going to make changes one meal at a time. So please be patient. It is far better than losing a few pounds quickly and gaining them right back for the hundredth time.

This is a good time to look over the food rankings (appendix E). Check out the Gold and Silver sections for some good breakfast ideas. It will also be a good idea to experiment with two or three new breakfast choices. Most people are not going to want to eat the same breakfast every day. It may also take a few tries before you find a few new and healthier breakfasts that you can enjoy on a regular basis.

Let's review some guidelines for making changes for meals and snacks:

GIUDELINES FOR MAKING MEAL

& SNACK SELECTION

The following examples are based on a 2,500-calorie (kcal.) per day diet that includes 3 meals and 2 snacks.

1. The average of each of the 3 meals should be approximately 625 calories or roughly 25% of the total caloric intake for the day. Individuals typically do not eat 3 meals of equal calories, but 625 calories should be the average. Each of the two snacks should equal roughly 250 calories or 12% of the total calories for the day. Needless to say, all the nutrient values (e.g., protein, fat, fiber, etc.) within the meal or snack should remain around 25% and 12% of the entire day respectively.

Example of the nutrient content for a Meal and Snack for a person eating 2,500 calories per day:

Nutrient	2,500 kcal. Day	One Meal (25%)	One Snack (12%)
Calories	2,500 kcal.	625 kcal.	300 kcal.
Carbohydrates	281–325 g	75 g	36 g
Protein	63-94 g	20 g	10 g
Total Fat	56-97 g	19 g	9 g

Saturated Fat	< 28 g	< 7 g	3 g
Trans Fat	*sparingly*	*sparingly*	*sparingly*
Cholesterol	<300 mg	*75 mg*	*36 mg*
Sodium	<2300 mg	*575 mg*	*275 mg*
Fiber	35 g	*9 g*	*4 g*
Sugar	<156 g	*40 g*	*15 g*
Fruit Serving	2–4 servings	*1 or more*	*1 or more*
Veggie Serving	3–5 servings	*1 or more*	*1 or more*

2. Try to balance each meal or snack with a combination of carbohydrates, protein, and fat. The purpose is to stabilize blood sugar levels and promote satiety until the next meal.

A quick review of the macronutrients:

- *Carbohydrates*—found in breads, cereals, bakery items, grains, candy, and starchy vegetables like potatoes, corn, and peas. Non-starchy vegetables like broccoli, cucumbers, tomatoes, and peppers have a minimal amount of carbohydrates.

- *Proteins*—includes meats such as red meat, poultry, and fish, although significant amounts of protein can also be found in eggs, peanut butter, dairy products, nuts, legumes (e.g., lentils), and soy products like tofu.

- *Fats*—mainly butter, margarine, and cooking oils, although significant amounts can be found in meats, dairy products, avocados, and nuts.

Keep in mind that many foods are a combination of one or more of the macronutrients. For example:

- **Milk** is a combination of carbohydrates, protein, and fat.

- **Nuts, cheese, and avocados** are a combination of fat and protein.
- **Pizza** is a combination of carbohydrates, protein, and fat.
- **Meats** contain varying amounts of protein and fat.
- **Legumes** are a combination of carbohydrates and protein.

3. Review the food rankings for help in choosing healthy meals and snacks. The general guidelines for the Gold, Silver, Bronze, and Zero-Value foods are as follows:

The main rationale for judging whether a food is Gold, Silver, Bronze, or Zero-Value is determined by the likelihood that the particular food will help or hinder the dieter in staying within his nutritional requirements for the day. Once again, a lower ranking implies that the food will make it mathematically more difficult for the dieter to stay within his recommended daily goal.

4. Read the selection tips that on the top of each food category in the food rankings.

5. Remember: The work you put in now will benefit you for the rest of your life. Spend the time now to find the nutrient content of the foods you eat on a regular basis. Look them up once and you will know them forever.

Let's check-out Fast-Food Freddy, Snack-Happy Steve, and Duck-Hook Harry to see what improvements they made to their breakfast choices.

Fast-Food Freddy

Freddy usually starts his day by throwing two Pop-Tarts into the toaster and opening a can of Diet Coke. Occasionally he would stop on his way to work at McDonald's or Dunkin Donuts.

After reviewing the food rankings he decided to improve his breakfast choices by switching from the Pop-Tarts, ranked as Bronze, to Kashi brand Frozen Waffles, which are ranked as Gold. The brand name for these waffles is Kashi, but any company with the same superior nutritional content would be fine. I am not promoting any companies or knocking others. I am only concerned with the nutritional content of the products.

Notice that these waffles have 8 grams of protein, 6 grams of fiber, 4 grams of sugar, and no saturated fat. This is a big improvement over the Pop-Tarts, which have 5 grams of protein, 1 gram of fiber, 33 grams of sugar, and 2 grams of saturated fat.

Freddy has also added orange juice for breakfast and is cutting down on his intake of Diet Coke.

Freddy will also experiment during the week with the addition of a shake or smoothie made with frozen fruit. Another option for Freddy is going to be the bodybuilding type shakes like Met-Rx or Myoplex, especially when he begins to weight train with more intensity during the off-season.

Snack-Happy Steve

Steve started most weekdays with a bowl of Cocoa Puffs cereal with whole milk and a cup of coffee with cream. He is going to switch to one of his wife's favorite cereals, which is Raisin Bran. He will also switch to her 2% milk and add a banana. He loves his coffee with cream and does not intend to give that up. The change in cereals has added 6 grams of protein and 13 grams of fiber.

More options for Steve include a bagel with low-fat cream cheese along with a bowl of fruit. Steve is also looking forward to a hot bowl of oatmeal during the colder months.

<u>Duck-Hook Harry</u>

Harry has become accustomed to starting each day with a hot breakfast from the coffee shop near his office. Harry has never prepared a meal in his life and does not intend to start now. He frequently ordered fried eggs with bacon along with the hash browns that he loves. Harry now continues to have his hash browns but now orders an egg white vegetable omelet. He has also made an effort to put as little butter as possible on his rye toast. Harry can easily add variety to his diet by ordering the many healthy selections on the menu, such as, oatmeal with banana, whole grain cereals, waffles, or pancakes.

STEP #4

What we want to do now is select a breakfast that you will eat other than your improved selections. This will be called your "not-so-healthy" selection. It may take time to completely give up the foods that you are accustomed to eating. You should not feel obligated to eat your improved breakfast every day of the week. The idea is to gradually change to a better diet. We also want to be able to compare the two breakfast selections (healthy and not-so-healthy) by filling out a scorecard for each of the two meals. One meal will be your new and improved healthy breakfast and the other will be the not-so-healthy selection. You will learn a lot by seeing in black and white just how these two meals compare. At the end of training camp, you will have completed two days of food choices onto a scorecard, and be able to compare your new and improved healthy scorecard and your not-so-healthy food scorecard. It is a great learning tool and is going to be an eye opening experience that you will never forget.

Let's take a look at what Freddy, Steve, and Harry selected for their second breakfast. The completed scorecards for the healthy and not-so-healthy breakfast and morning snacks of Fast-Food Freddy are listed in Tables 7-1 and 7-2. The completed scorecards for the healthy and not-so-healthy breakfast and morning snacks of Snack-Happy Steve are listed in Tables 7-3 and 7-4, and Duck-Hook Harry's are listed in Tables 7-5 and 7-6.

Fast-Food Freddy

Freddy is going to select his old breakfast of Pop-Tarts as his not-so-healthy selection. He may also have an occasional Egg McMuffin if he happens to be near a McDonald's on the weekend.

Snack-Happy Steve

Steve is going to use the not-so-healthy scorecard to analyze his old diet. He really wants to know how bad he was actually eating. He will select his Cocoa Puffs breakfast for the not-so-healthy scorecard.

Duck-Hook Harry

Harry is going to select his bacon and eggs breakfast for his not-so-healthy selection. That is the breakfast that he ate most often before starting training camp.

STEP #5

The next dietary change we are going to make this week is with your morning snack. Once again, it is a good idea to review the Gold and Silver sections of the food rankings and find a snack that is healthier than the one you are currently having. It may take a few tries before you find a couple of snacks that are satisfying. Chances are good that you will be buying some foods that you end up not liking. That can be expected. But it is worth it when you find a new and improved snack that you can enjoy for the rest of your life. Remember, it takes a lot of work to change old habits. That is why we are devoting an entire week to changing one meal and one snack. With each subsequent dieting cycle you will be able to make more improvements until your diet is not only healthy but also satisfying.

Let's check in with our guys and see how they are handling this step:

Fast-Food Freddy

Freddy has his morning snack at the office each day. Usually that consisted of a Danish, pastry, or coffee cake. Not being a coffee drinker, he washes it down with a Diet Coke. Freddy never thought that these snacks were a good choice, but figured, "What the hell, they're right in front of me." Freddy decided to switch to a Clif brand energy bar. He also looks forward to his Diet Coke since he is no longer has one for breakfast.

Snack-Happy Steve

Steve loves his chocolate donuts, but is ready to experiment with some healthier snacks. He is now going to have a bran muffin or a small bagel with some low-fat cream cheese and a fresh glass of orange juice.

Note that Steve and Freddy are eating more calories during the morning than they did before starting this diet. This is fine because it will sustain their energy throughout the day and reduce the likelihood of them overeating during the rest of the day.

Duck-Hook Harry

Harry usually has a big breakfast and is too busy to stop for a morning snack. But when he does, it is normally a piece of cheese Danish that he washes down with his trademark black coffee. He will switch to two small oatmeal cookies.

STEP #6

Now we are going to select a second snack. Similar to what we just did with breakfast, we need to pick another snack for the one or two days that you don't feel like having your new and improved selection. Most likely, you won't want to eat your new healthier snack every single day. Therefore, your second selection will be the not-so-healthy snack that you are currently eating or another selection all together. Some people are inclined to review the Bronze section of the food rankings to find an appropriate selection. Many people wish to eliminate all foods from the Zero-Value section right from the start. Again, the choice is yours. If you need a snack from the Zero-Value section in order not to feel deprived, then by all means, go right ahead. But do try your best to refrain from all Zero-Value foods.

Let's check in with our guys and see how they are handling this step:

Fast-Food Freddy

Freddy figures that once a week he will eat whatever coffee cake or pastry that is in the snack room at work.

Snack-Happy Steve

Steve is still going to have his chocolate donut every now and then.

<u>Duck-Hook Harry</u>

Similar to Freddy, Harry will indulge in whatever bakery item that is sitting around the office. Harry does not anticipate this happening more than once every week or two.

STEP #7

We are going to start filling out two different scorecards. One will be for your healthy day, and the other will be the not-so-healthy day. Make sure you write the words "healthy" and "not-so-healthy" on the top of your scorecards.

Record your healthy breakfast selections along with all the nutritional information onto one scorecard. The other scorecard will consist of your not-so-healthy food choices. The not-so-healthy day would most likely consist of foods that are eaten on weekends or other foods that are not quite ready to give up.

If you haven't done so already, a sample scorecard can be photocopied from appendix B or downloaded from http://www.rayoflife.com. Each scorecard will have enough space to input the nutritional information for one meal and a snack. It will take three individual scorecards to record the information for one day. The information from the three scorecards (appendix B) will then be transcribed onto a form titled Scorecard—Totals for the Day (appendix C) or downloaded from http://www.rayoflife.com.

Keep in mind that we are trying to get approximate values for the nutritional content of two typical days of eating. One day represents a healthy day of eating, while the other is a not-so-healthy day of eating. The purpose is for you to see in black and white the nutritional differences between the two. Most likely, your diet will range somewhere between these healthy and not-so-healthy days. By knowing the two extremes of your diet, you will be able to estimate various days of eating for the rest of your life, without doing all the calculations. You will be able to say to yourself, "Hey, today I'm eating better than that healthy day of eating that I recorded." Or you may say, "Oh no, today I'm eating worse than my not-so-healthy day."

Food choices vary constantly and it is difficult to get exact measurements of what you are eating. But we can learn more than enough to improve our understanding of the foods that we eat every single day. It just isn't right for a sports-minded male to know everything about sports and nothing about the foods he eats.

As I have already mentioned, the completed scorecards for the healthy and not-so-healthy breakfast and morning snacks of Fast-Food Freddy are listed in Tables 7-1 and 7-2. The completed scorecards for the healthy and not-so-healthy breakfast and morning snacks of Snack-Happy Steve are listed in Tables 7-3 and 7-4, and Duck-Hook Harry's are listed in Tables 7-5 and 7-6.

Table 7 – 1: Scorecard

Name: _Freddy_ Date: _Jan. 4-10, 2010_ Dieting Cycle: _1_ Week#: _1_ .
Type of Day: _Healthy_ Calorie Goal: _2,765_ Activity Level: _Light_ .

Food Item	Amount	Calories	Carbohydrate	Protein	Total Fat	Saturated Fat	Trans Fat	Cholesterol	Sodium	Fiber	Sugar	Fruit Serving	Veggie Serving
Meal: Breakfast													
Waffles – Kashi/Go-Lean	2 ea	170	33	8	3	0	0	0	300	6	4	0	0
Butter	1 tbsp	50	1	0	6	4	0	15	95	0	0	0	0
Maple Syrup	1 oz	104	27	0	0	0	0	0	4	0	24	0	0
Orange Juice	12 oz	186	48	0	0	0	0	0	49	0	47	1.5	0
Snack: Morning													
Clif Bar - almond	1 ea	231	38	10	5	1	0	0	139	5	20	0	0
Diet Coke	12 oz	1	0	0	0	0	0	0	6	0	0	0	0
Total:		742	147	18	14	5	0	15	593	11	95	1.5	0

Table 7 – 2: Scorecard

Name: *Freddy* Date: *Jan 4-10, 2010* Dieting Cycle: _1_ Week#: _1_ .
Type of Day: *Not so Healthy* Calorie Goal: _2,765_ Activity Level: _Light_.

Food Item	Amount	Calories	Carbohydrate	Protein	Total Fat	Saturated Fat	Trans Fat	Cholesterol	Sodium	Fiber	Sugar	Fruit Serving	Veggie Serving
Meal: *Breakfast*													
Pop Tart - cherry	2 pc	409	74	5	11	2	-	0	440	1	33	-	-
Diet Coke	12 oz	1	0	0	0	0	0	0	6	0	0	-	-
Snack: *Morning*													
Coffee Cake - Cinnamon	1 pc	178	30	3	5	1	-	27	236	1	17	-	-
Diet Coke	12 oz	1	0	0	0	0	0	0	6	0	0	-	-
Total:		589	104	8	16	3	0	27	688	2	50	0	0

Table 7 – 3: Scorecard

Name: _Steve_ Date: _Jan. 4-10, 2010_ Dieting Cycle: _1_ Week #: _1_ .
Type of Day: _Healthy_ Calorie Goal: _3,049_ Activity Level: _Light_ .

Food Item	Amount	Calories	Carbohydrate	Protein	Total Fat	Saturated Fat	Trans Fat	Cholesterol	Sodium	Fiber	Sugar	Fruit Serving	Veggie Serving
Meal: _Breakfast_													
Raisin Bran Cereal	2 c	380	92	8	2	0	-	0	600	16	38	-	-
2% Milk	1 c	122	11	8	5	3	0	20	100	0	11	-	-
Banana – whole	1 ea	105	27	1	0	0	0	0	1	3	14	1	0
Coffee	2 c	5	0	1	0	0	0	0	9	0	0	0	0
Cream	1 oz	39	1	1	3	2	0	11	1	0	0	0	0
Snack: _Morning_													
Bran Muffin w/ raisins	1 ea	106	19	2	3	0	-	6	178	3	5	0	0
Low-fat cream cheese	2 tbsp	69	2	3	5	3	-	17	89	0	0	0	0
Orange Juice	1 c	112	26	2	0	0	0	0	2	0	21	1	0
Total:		938	178	26	18	8	0	54	980	22	89	2	0

Table 7 – 4: Scorecard

Name: *Steve* Date: *Jan. 4-10, 2010* Dieting Cycle: *1* Week#: *1* .
Type of Day: *Not so Healthy* Calorie Goal: *3,049* Activity Level: *Light* .

Food Item	Amount	Calories	Carbohydrate	Protein	Total Fat	Saturated Fat	Trans Fat	Cholesterol	Sodium	Fiber	Sugar	Fruit Serving	Veggie Serving
Meal: *Breakfast*													
Cocoa Puffs cereal	2 c	240	52	2	3	0	0	0	320	3	28	-	-
Whole Milk	1 c	146	11	8	8	5	0	24	98	0	11	-	-
Coffee-brewed	2 c	5	0	1	0	0	0	0	9	0	0	-	-
Cream - half and half	1 oz	39	1	1	3	2	0	11	12	0	0	-	-
Snack: *Morning*													
Chocolate Donut	1 ea	250	25	3	15	5	-	0	270	2	12	-	-
Coffee-brewed	2 c	5	0	1	0	0	0	0	9	0	0	-	-
Cream-half and half	1 oz	39	1	1	3	2	0	11	12	0	0	-	-
Total:		724	90	17	32	14	0	46	730	5	51	0	0

Name: *Harry* Date: *Jan. 4-10, 2010* Dieting Cycle: *1* Week#: *1* .
Type of Day: *Healthy* Calorie Goal: *2482* Activity Level: *Light* .

Food Item	Amount	Calories	Carbohydrate	Protein	Total Fat	Saturated Fat	Trans Fat	Cholesterol	Sodium	Fiber	Sugar	Fruit Serving	Veggie Serving
Meal: *Breakfast*													
Egg white omelet w/veggies	1 serv	93	6	15	0	0	0	0	224	1	4	-	0
Olive Oil - cooking	1 tbsp	119	0	0	14	2	-	0	0	0	0	-	-
Hash Browns	2 ea	200	30	4	8	2	-	0	400	4	0	-	1
Rye Bread	1 slice	80	15	3	1	0	-	0	210	2	1	-	-
Butter	1 tsp	33	0	0	4	2	0	10	27	0	0	-	-
Snack: *Morning*													
Oatmeal Cookie	2 ea	180	30	2	7	2	-	10	100	2	14	-	-
Coffee	8 oz.	2	0	0	0	0	0	0	5	0	0	-	-
Total:		709	81	24	34	8	0	20	971	9	19	0	1

Table 7 – 6: Scorecard

Name: _Harry_ Date: _Jan 4-10, 2010_ Dieting Cycle: _1_ Week#: _1_.
Type of Day: _Not so-Healthy_ Calorie Goal: _2,482_ Activity Level: _Light._

Food Item	Amount	Calories	Carbohydrate	Protein	Total Fat	Saturated Fat	Trans Fat	Cholesterol	Sodium	Fiber	Sugar	Fruit Serving	Veggie Serving
Meal:													
Breakfast													
Fried Eggs in vegetable oil	3 ea	363	0	19	32	7	-	589	290	0	0	-	-
Bacon- pan-fried	3 strip	308	1	21	24	8	0	63	1317	0	0	-	-
Rye Bread	1 slice	120	25	4	1	0	-	0	430	3	2	-	-
Butter	1 tbsp	100	0	0	11	7	-	30	81	0	0	-	-
Hash Browns	1 serv	136	13	1	9	2	2	0	289	2	0	-	0
Coffee	8 oz	2	0	0	0	0	0	0	5	0	0	-	-
Snack:													
Morning													
Cheese Danish	1 serv	266	26	6	16	5	-	11	320	1	5	-	-
Coffee	8 oz	2	0	0	0	0	0	0	5	0	0	-	-
Total:		1297	65	51	93	29	2	693	2737	6	7	0	0

STEP #8

The last thing we are going to do this week is to learn a little bit about the Nutrition Facts food label that is on the package of most foods. Many of the foods that you eat will not be listed in the food rankings section; therefore you will need to get the information from the package.

An example of a Nutrition Facts food label is listed below in Table 7-7.

Table 7-7

Nutrition Facts

Serving Size 1 cup (228g)
Servings Per Container 2

Amount Per Serving	
Calories 250	Calories from Fat 110

	% Daily Value*
Total Fat 12g	18%
Saturated Fat 3g	15%
Trans Fat 1.5g	
Cholesterol 30mg	10%
Sodium 470mg	20%
Total Carbohydrate 31g	10%
Dietary Fiber 0g	0%
Sugars 5g	
Protein 5g	

Vitamin A	4%
Vitamin C	2%
Calcium	20%
Iron	4%

* Percent Daily Values are based on a 2,000 calorie diet. Your Daily Values may be higher or lower depending on your calorie needs:

	Calories:	2,000	2,500
Total Fat	Less than	65g	80g
Sat Fat	Less than	20g	25g
Cholesterol	Less than	300mg	300mg
Sodium	Less than	2,400mg	2,400mg
Total Carbohydrate		300g	375g
Dietary Fiber		25g	30g

The first thing you want to do when reading the food label is to figure out how many servings of the food you are going to be eating. Look at the top of the label for the serving size, then immediately look at how many servings are in one package. In the case of the label in Table 7-7, there are 2 serving sizes in one package (container). One serving (one cup is this case) is 250 calories. Therefore, if you were to eat the whole package (which is very likely) you would be consuming 500 calories. It goes without saying that all the other amounts would also be doubled as well. Not exactly rocket science, but I thought that I should mention it.

In order to complete your scorecard, you will simply record the information from the package onto your scorecard. You will also have to determine on your own whether the food you are consuming is a fruit or a vegetable and how many servings of a fruit or vegetable it contains. I have complete confidence that you will be able to tell a fruit from a vegetable, but determining the number of servings may be more difficult. I will explain shortly how that can be easily done on the Internet. There is no need to freak-out if you are not sure whether ketchup or french fries count as a vegetable. What we are trying to do is increase the intake of fruit (fresh, frozen, dried, or juiced), and healthy vegetables in the form of green salads, peppers, tomatoes, broccoli, squash, sweet potatoes, baked potatoes, and other similar good stuff.

Another important feature of the food label is the "% Daily Value" listed in the right-hand column. The percentage listed in that column is the percentage that one serving of the particular food has in relation to the amount required for one day, assuming a two-thousand-calorie diet. In other words, the one serving of the product in Table 7-7 contains 18% of the total fat that is required for the whole day. If you consumed the entire package (two servings), then you would have consumed 36% of the fat that is recommended for one day, if you were on a two-thousand-calorie diet. A general rule of thumb is that a %Daily Value over 20 percent is considered high, while a % Daily Value that is 5 percent or less is considered low. Are we all clear on that? Good.

There are more options for you to get the nutritional information that you need. Perhaps the fastest and easiest way is to use the Internet. The Food and Nutrition Information Center of the USDA has a Web site that makes it relatively easy to find the nutritional information on just about any food. The Web site address is: http://fnic.nal.usda.gov/
Here are the steps once you enter the homepage:

1. On the homepage, click *Food Composition* on the sidebar on the left side of the page.
2. Once on the *Food Composition* page, click on *USDA Nutrient Data Laboratory* on the top, middle portion of the screen.
3. Next, in the middle of the page, click on the first bulleted heading: *Online searchable database of foods*. This will get you to the USDA Nutrient Data Laboratory.
4. You are now ready to input your food choices. But first I suggest that you click HELP to get a better understanding of how to search for the foods. Note: this Web site lists more nutrient information than you will need. Just take the information that you need to complete your scorecard. Also notice that instead of using the term "Calories" they use the term "Energy" listed as kcal—i.e., kilocalorie—units. Do not be alarmed, these terms are synonymous.
5. There are other valuable links that can found on the *Food Composition* page. On the right sidebar you will find a link titled *Additional Resources*. Here you will be led to three very valuable links:

    1. *CalorieKing.com* Food Database—Nutritional information for over 45,000 generic and brand name foods (including over 260 fast-food chains)

with a wide range of nutrient data and information.

2.   *Fast Food Guide* — Nutritional information for many fast food restaurants including: Arby's, Burger King, Carl's Jr., Domino's Pizza, Dunkin Donuts, Jack-In-The-Box, Kentucky Fried Chicken, McDonald's, Subway, Taco Bell, Wendy's and more.

3.   *MyFood-a-pedia* — Provides quick access to food information including food groups, calories, and comparison of two foods. This is the site that you can use to determine the number of fruit and vegetable servings that are in the food that you select.

You can learn all you ever want to know about food from these Web sites. Spend some time navigating through the enormous amount of information provided by the USDA and its many links. You paid for these sites with your tax dollars, so you might as well use them. It really is a shame that they are not promoted or advertised on a larger scale. Please, do yourself a big favor and check them out.

STEP #9

Select two mornings that you will be weighing yourself. You will be weighing yourself two times a week for the rest of your life. Nothing is going to keep you more focused and out of denial than weighing yourself twice a week. As I have already mentioned, weighing yourself should not be a traumatic event. Just jump on the damn scale. Your weight *is* what it *is*. You need to know how your body weight fluctuates according to your actions. It is certainly OK to indulge in food or drink, but you need to be man enough to see what it is doing to you. If you know the nutritional content of the foods you are indulging in and you know what it is doing to your weight, then you can make an informed decision on whether you want to continue or not. Sometimes, just knowing the facts is all you need to make the right decision. In either case, it is another choice that only you can make.

STEP #10

Thank goodness that sports-minded males already know how to work out (exercise). Therefore, the suggestions that I make will focus mostly on the proper frequency, duration, and intensity of your workouts and not delve into the type of exercise you are doing. During the first four weeks of training camp, we will be focused mostly on the frequency of your workouts. If you are not exercising at all, then it is time to start with a minimum of three times a week. The goal is to exercise in the neighborhood of three hours per week at a low-to-moderate intensity. If you are already exercising more than three hours per week, you can continue your normal routine, but at a low-to-moderate intensity. What you don't want to do is start out like a bat out of hell. Your primary concern during this time is to improve the quality of the food that you are eating, not to obsess about reducing calories or working out like a madman. There will be plenty of time in the near future to reduce calories and to work out intensely, but not now.

Here's what Fast-Food Freddy, Snack-Happy Steve, and Duck-Hook Harry are going to do for exercise:

Fast-Food Freddy

Freddy hasn't been working out at all. His plan is to start out very slow and begin to carve out a few time slots during the week for exercise. Freddy doesn't mind working out and realizes that the hardest part is going to be finding the time to incorporate exercise back into his schedule. He is going to dust off his gym membership card and head to the gym every Tuesday and Thursday night after work. Freddy will start his workout at the gym with twenty to thirty minutes of cardio followed by thirty minutes of weight training with moderate resistance in a up-tempo, circuit training type pace. Freddy will then cool down with some stretching. He will add a third workout with his girlfriend on the weekends. They have roller bladed, hiked, and biked in the past and are excited to start again. He was glad to know that exercising at a low-to-moderate intensity is the way to go for now. In the past he always went all-out and then petered out soon after.

Snack-Happy Steve

Steve's wife belongs to a health club, but Steve has never been a health club type of guy. He has done some jogging in the past and completed a few 10K races about seven years ago. Steve, as a salesperson, is accustomed to being goal oriented. As a source of motivation, he has committed to run a 10K race that is scheduled in six months. He has no idea what his time will be, but his goal is to complete it without having to walk. In the good old days, he ran at an eight-minute-per-mile pace. But that was seven years and forty pounds ago.

Wisely, Steve is going to start his exercise routine by walking thirty minutes, three mornings a week, before his phone starts ringing off the hook. Each night he will get additional activity by playing catch with his boys or shooting a few baskets. He will also lift a few weights in the basement with an old weight set that is currently covered with junk. He will eventually get his stationary bike fixed to add variety to his routine and have a bad weather option.

Duck-Hook Harry

When Harry sets his mind to something he usually goes all-out. He is well aware that he knows nothing about exercise and therefore will begin to research the topic extensively. Friends of his have recommended everything from Aikido to Yoga, but he is having a difficult time deciding. Harry finally decided to join the health club near his office and work out three days a week during lunch. Harry loves people and has no reservations at all about trying the many classes that the club offers. He plans to take advantage of the many healthy dishes and smoothies offered at the club's cafe.

Chapter 8:
Training Camp—Week Two

STEP #1

During week one you selected a healthy breakfast and morning snack, along with a not-so-healthy breakfast and snack. You also took the time to record the nutritional information of these meals and snacks onto your scorecards. You will now do the same for your lunch and afternoon snack.

For week two, the primary objective will be the improvement of your lunch selections and afternoon snack. Similar to your breakfast changes, these alterations can be a minor tweaking of your current lunch or a complete overhaul. For example, an appropriate challenge for one person may be switching from a cheeseburger and large fries to a hamburger with small fries. Another person may decide to change his customary lunch from a cheeseburger and fries to a sandwich of whole grain bread with turkey, tuna, or chicken. Beneficial changes can also be made with your beverage selections. Cutting back on soda is a great place to start. As with breakfast, you will need to select a few new lunch choices to provide variety to your diet. Only you can know which changes are appropriate for you. Keep in mind that it is easy to plan major changes on Sunday night when your stomach is full and you are relaxed and rested. But more often than not, these "pie in the sky" changes cannot be sustained for an extended period of time or in times of stress. Once again, the tendency will be to do too much, too soon. Keep this in mind when you are planning your changes; you want to do enough to feel good about yourself by meeting the challenge, but meeting the challenge shouldn't create a sense of drudgery. Think about the effort it would take to learn to play golf or tennis. Typically, as you are improving your game, you'll go through alternating times of encouragement and frustration. Well, learning to eat better is no different. The idea is to continue at a pace that fosters more encouragement while minimizing the frustration. Only you will be able to determine the proper pace and appropriate challenge.

The goal at the end of the week is for you to have two or more new improved lunch choices that you can implement into your diet without a sense of deprivation. By the way, you will continue to eat your new and improved healthy breakfast and snack at least five times a week.

Let's check in on the guys to see how they are handling this step:

Fast-Food Freddy

Freddy is going to start week two by switching from his Quarter Pounder with cheese and large fries to a chicken sandwich at Wendy's. He is going to do his best not to have a Diet Coke with lunch. If he does, then he won't have one during his afternoon break. His overall goal is to cut back from four Diet Cokes a day to only two. For another improved lunch, Freddy will visit Subway for a turkey sandwich (easy on the mayo) or another of its healthier choices.

Snack-Happy Steve

Steve has gotten into the habit of having deli meat sandwiches, potato chips, and a Coke every day for lunch. He is going to start having more peanut butter and jelly sandwiches, which he loves. Another improvement he will make is having corn tortilla chips instead of potato chips. He will also switch from regular Coke to Diet Coke and add an apple. His switch to Diet Coke is a good example of why each person's diet needs to be personalized. Steve is going to be adding a Diet Coke for lunch while Freddy is trying to remove it. It's a good example of how one size does not fit all when it comes to dieting. Eventually both guys will cut it out of their diets, one step at a time.

Other options for Steve include a tuna sandwich on whole grain bread or a turkey salad plate made with leftover fresh turkey breast.

Duck-Hook Harry

Harry often has lunch meetings at the better restaurants in town. A typical choice of his would be Fettuccini Alfredo, along with a few dinner rolls and a glass of wine. Harry is going to begin week two with a more sensible lunch selection like Pasta Primavera, a small salad with balsamic vinaigrette dressing (on the side). If he does have a dinner roll, he will try to use as little butter as possible. He is also going to have his wine in the evening and enjoy some sparkling water during lunch.

STEP #2

Now is the time to select a lunch other than your healthier selections. This will be considered your not-so-healthy lunch. This, once again, will be a lunch that you will have occasionally or on weekends. As you know by now, your healthy choices do not have to be eaten every day, unless you choose to do so.

Now let's see what the guys select as their not-so-healthy lunches:

Fast-Food Freddy

Freddy doesn't plan on totally abandoning McDonald's. Now and then he will visit Mickey Dee's for some of his old favorites like the Quarter Pounder and fries.

Snack-Happy Steve

Steve will look forward to having a ham and cheese sandwich on the weekend. When he does, he will still make improvements by substituting whole grain bread for his customary white bread. He will go easy on the mayonnaise and limit himself to only a few potato chips.

Duck-Hook Harry

Harry loves heavy dishes and dairy products. He will continue to eat Fettuccini Alfredo, grilled cheese sandwiches, and veal parmesan, but not nearly as often.

STEP #3

Now is the time to select a healthier afternoon snack. A healthier snack can be selected from the Gold and Silver sections of the food rankings. You may also find it helpful to browse the supermarket or health food store for something that looks appealing. Make sure that you analyze the Nutrition Facts food label to be certain that it is indeed a healthy snack. The Nutrition Facts food label of any item that you find should resemble those of the snack items listed in the Gold and Silver sections of the food rankings. Make special note of the amounts of trans fat, saturated fat, and sodium that are contained in many snack items.

Let's check in on the guys:

Fast-Food Freddy

Freddy has gotten into the habit of getting a candy bar from the vending machine as his afternoon snack. He is now going to switch to a trail mix that includes a lot of dried fruit. Freddy has always liked trail mix, but has been too lazy to do the shopping for this and other healthy foods.

Snack-Happy Steve

Steve has been a cake and cookie monster in the afternoons. Toward the end of the day, his energy has been low and his stress levels high. Normally he would head straight to the cabinet high above the refrigerator that stores all the goodies like cupcakes and Twinkies. He realizes that this habit has got to change and is now going to start having one of his wife's favorites — low-fat yogurt topped with Grape-Nuts. He actually likes it, and will try to change his perception that this is a girlie snack.

Duck-Hook Harry

Harry has never been a snacker. The only time Harry has snacks is when he is out on the golf course. He will start to carry a nonmelting energy bar in his golf bag to help keep his blood sugar stable. Clif Bars are perfect for Harry. They come in many varieties and do not melt on hot days. When it comes to bars, everyone will have to experiment. Clif is one brand that I know is good, but there are others.

STEP #4

You will now select a not-so-healthy snack for the times that you don't feel like being so healthy. On these occasions, you may choose a snack that you still crave. Feeling deprived is not the way to go. Keep in mind that you may also find that you no longer enjoy some of your favorite unhealthy snacks. Often, your new attitude and knowledge of foods will turn you off to the foods that you once loved. You may also find that you feel like crap after eating unhealthy foods after your body becomes accustomed to eating better.

Let's take a look at how the guys are handling this step:

Fast-Food Freddy

Freddy will have his favorite Snickers bar from time to time.

Snack-Happy Steve

For the time being, Steve is going to have the occasional cupcake.

Duck-Hook Harry

Harry doesn't normally snack in the afternoon. He likes his three square meals a day. Harry may be one of those guys who are better off eating only three times a day.

STEP #5

Now you need to record the nutritional information of your improved lunch and snack onto your scorecard. Similar to last week, you will fill out one scorecard for your healthy lunch and afternoon snack, and a second scorecard for your not-so-healthy selections

Examples of the healthy and not-so-healthy lunches and afternoon snacks of Freddy, Steve, and Harry can be found in Tables 8-1 and 8-2 (Freddy), 8-3 and 8-4 (Steve), and 8-5 and 8-6 (Harry).

Table 8 – 1: Scorecard

Name: _Freddy_ Date: _Jan 11-17, 2010_ Dieting Cycle: _1_ Week#: _2_
Type of Day: _Healthy_ Calorie Goal: _2,765_ Activity Level: _Light_

Food Item	Amount	Calories	Carbohydrate	Prtein	Total Fat	Saturated Fat	Trans Fat	Cholsterol	Sodium	Fiber	Sugar	Fruit Serving	Veggie Serving
Meal: *Lunch*													
Chicken Grilled Sandwich-Wendy's	1 ea	300	36	24	7	2	0	55	740	2	8	0	0
Baked Potato-Wendy's	1 ea	310	72	7	0	0	0	0	25	7	5	0	2
Butter	1 serv	50	1	0	6	4	0	15	95	0	0	0	0
Water	12 oz	0	0	0	0	0	0	0	11	0	0	0	0
Salsa	1 serv	30	6	1	0	0	0	0	440	0	4	0	0
Snack: *Afternoon*													
Bar-Trail Mix/Fruit & Nut	1 ea	140	25	3	4	1	0	0	95	2	13	0	0
Diet Coke	12 oz	1	0	0	0	0	0	0	6	0	0	0	0
Raisins-small box	1 ea	129	34	1	0	0	0	0	5	2	25	1	0
Total:		960	174	36	17	7	0	70	1417	13	55	1	2

Table 8 – 2: Scorecard

Name: *Freddy* Date: *Jan. 11-17, 2010* Dieting Cycle: *1* Week#: *2.*
Type of Day: *Not so Healthy* Calorie Goal: *2,482* Activity Level: *Light.*

Food Item	Amount	Calories	Carbohydrate	Prtein	Total Fat	Saturated Fat	Trans Fat	Cholsterol	Sodium	Fiber	Sugar	Fruit Serving	Veggie Serving
Meal: *Lunch*													
Quarter Pounder w/cheese	1 ea	513	40	29	28	11	2	94	1152	3	10	-	0
Large Fries	1 ea	576	70	6	31	6	8	0	332	7	0	-	2
Diet Coke	12 oz.	1	0	0	0	0	0	0	6	0	0	0	0
Snack: *Afternoon*													
Snickers Bar	1 ea	539	69	9	27	10	0	15	279	3	57	-	-
Total:		1629	179	44	86	27	10	109	1769	13	67	0	2

Table 3 – 3: Scorecard

Name: *Steve* Date: *Jan 11-17, 2010* Dieting Cycle: *1* Week#: *2*

Type of Day: *Healthy* Calorie Goal: *3,049* Activity Level: *Light.*

Food Item	Amount	Calories	Carbohydrate	Prtein	Total Fat	Saturated Fat	Trans Fat	Cholesterol	Sodium	Fiber	Sugar	Fruit Serving	Veggie Serving
Meal: *Lunch*													
Peanut Butter/Jelly - whole wheat bread	1 ea	398	51	13	17	4	-	0	465	5	17	-	-
Chips - tortilla/blue	1 serv	110	22	3	2	0	-	0	140	2	0	-	-
Apple -medium	1 ea	72	19	0	0	0	0	0	1	3	14	1	0
Diet Coke	12 oz	1	0	0	0	0	0	0	6	0	0	0	0
Snack: *Afternoon*													
Fruit Yogurt	8 oz	231	43	10	2	2	-	9	132	0	43	-	-
Grape Nuts	2 tbsp	52	12	2	0	0	-	0	88	1	2	-	-
Total:		864	147	27	21	6	0	9	832	11	76	1	0

Table 8 – 4: Scorecard

Name: _Steve_ Date: _Jan 11-17, 2010_ Dieting Cycle: _1_ Week#: _2_.
Type of Day: _Not so Healthy_ Calorie Goal: _3,049_ Activity Level: _Light_

Food Item	Amount	Calories	Carbohydrate	Protein	Total Fat	Saturated Fat	Trans Fat	Cholesterol	Sodium	Fiber	Sugar	Fruit Serving	Veggie Serving
Meal:							*Lunch*						
Baked Ham - lunch meat	4 slice	80	2	16	1	0	-	40	1220	0	2	-	-
Swiss cheese	2 slice	220	0	16	18	10	-	60	100	0	0	-	-
Bread -White	2 slice	130	23	4	2	1	-	0	260	1	3	-	-
Coke	12 oz	180	46	0	0	0	0	-	67	0	46	-	-
Potato Chips	1 serv	155	14	2	11	3	-	0	149	1	0	-	1
Snack:							*Afternoon*						
Chocolate Cup Cake	1 ea	103	18	1	3	1	1	3	130	1	13	-	-
Milk- Whole	1 c	146	11	8	8	5	0	24	98	0	11	-	-
Total:		1014	114	47	43	20	1	127	2024	3	75	-	1

Table 8 – 5: Scorecard

Name: _Harry_ Date: _Jan. 11-17, 2010_ Dieting Cycle: _1_ Week#: _2_ .
Type of Day: _Healthy_ Calorie Goal: _2,482_ Activity Level: _Light_

Food Item	Amount	Calories	Carbohydrate	Protein	Total Fat	Saturated Fat	Trans Fat	Cholesterol	Sodium	Fiber	Sugar	Fruit Serving	Veggie Serving
Meal:									_Lunch_				
Pasta Primavera	1 serv	250	38	9	7	4	-	20	730	3	9	-	-
Dinner Roll	1 ea	133	22	5	3	1	-	2	230	1	2	-	-
Butter	1 tsp	33	0	0	4	2	0	10	27	0	0	-	-
Salad Dressing-balsamic	2 tbsp	80	3	0	8	0	0	0	230	0	2	-	-
Salad-tomato/cucumber/crouton	2 c	69	14	3	0	0	0	0	65	3	4	-	2
Snack:									_Afternoon_				
Total:		565	77	17	22	7	0	32	1282	7	17	-	2

Table 8 – 6: Scorecard

Name: *Harry* Date: *Jan 11-17, 2010* Dieting Cycle: *1* Week#: *1*.
Type of Day: *Not so Healthy* Calorie Goal: *2,482* Activity Level: *Light*.

Food Item	Amount	Calories	Carbohydrate	Protein	Total Fat	Saturated Fat	Trans Fat	Cholesterol	Sodium	Fiber	Sugar	Fruit Serving	Veggie Serving
Meal: *Lunch*													
Fettuccini Alfredo	1 serv	518	77	19	15	6	-	139	2195	-	-	-	-
Dinner Roll	2 ea	267	45	9	6	1	-	3	461	2	5	-	-
Butter	1 tbsp	100	4	0	11	7	0	30	81	0	0	-	-
Wine- Merlot	5 oz	123	4	0	0	0	0	-	6	0	1	-	-
Snack:													
Total:		1008	130	28	32	14	0	172	2743	2	6	0	0

Allow me to repeat; at the end of the three weeks you will have completed one scorecard with the information for your healthy breakfast and morning snack, a second scorecard with the information for your healthy lunch and afternoon snack, and a third one recording the nutritional information of your healthy dinner and dessert and/or evening snack. The totals of the three scorecards will then be transcribed onto the form titled, Scorecard – Totals for the Day (appendix C). You will also have another set of scorecards for your not-so-healthy meals and snacks. The totals of your not-so-healthy scorecards will also be transcribed onto the form titled, Scorecard – Totals for the Day. On this form you will be able to view the nutritional content of a complete day and analyze how the totals of your meals and snacks compare to the recommended dietary guidelines. You will also be able to compare how your healthy day compares to your not-so-healthy day. These calculations will be etched into your brain for the rest of your life.

STEP #6

Continue to exercise at least three times a week. Remember that the primary focus of week two is still the improvement of your food choices. Exercise has a better chance of becoming a natural part of your life if you make it challenging but still fun.

STEP #7

Continue weighing yourself on the same two mornings. Do not start altering the days that you weigh yourself according to whether you think you have lost weight. Don't be overly concerned about weight loss after only two weeks. Don't talk yourself into quitting if you haven't lost weight. We are all at the weights that we deserve. It is what it is. Having a hissy fit isn't going to help. Just stick with the program. The weight *will* come off. Never as fast as we would like, but it will come off.

Chapter 9:
Training Camp — Week Three

STEP #1

During week three, you will be making improvements to your dinner, dessert, and evening snack. You will begin by making improvements to your dinner choices. Keep in mind that dinner provides the best opportunity to add vegetables to your diet. By vegetables, I mean a variety of vegetables like carrots, green beans, potatoes, yams, corn, peas, squash, broccoli, cauliflower, and green leafy lettuce. You can easily get your recommended servings of vegetables by consuming mounds of french fries. But that is not what we are after. What we are looking for is an increase in the servings of healthy vegetables.

I'm certain that there are guys out there that respond to the thought of vegetables with a resounding, "Yuck!" Well, I won't bore you with all the benefits of vegetables, but I will say that vegetables and fruits will start tasting much better when you stop eating so much crap. The taste of fruit and vegetables can't compete with the contaminating flavors of the overly sugary and salty foods. As long as your taste buds are contaminated by inferior foods, you will continue to crave them. This is not much different from a cigarette smoker craving another cigarette. Not respecting the addictive power of inferior foods is a big-time mistake. Furthermore, you can easily regain your innate desire for natural foods, if you are willing to do the work necessary to gradually break old habits.

Generally speaking, your dinners will consist of the following categories:

PROTEIN: such as beef, pork, poultry, lamb, cheese, fish, beans, and tofu.

GRAINS: pasta, rice, bread.

STARCHY VEGETABLES: potatoes, corn, peas, yams, and squash.

NON STARCHY VEGETABLES: broccoli, cauliflower, carrots, lettuce, tomatoes, green beans, celery, and cucumber.

A common mistake is eating too much protein along with a grain and/or starchy vegetable, while ignoring the non starchy vegetables. Examples would be a dinner consisting of a cheeseburger with fries (protein, grain, and starchy vegetable), pizza (protein and grain), or a chicken burrito with rice (protein and grain). You get the idea. I know it doesn't sound very manly, but you got to start eating more non starchy vegetables, if you haven't already. These healthy foods will begin to decontaminate your taste buds. Eventually, even vegetables will taste great. I promise. Besides, they contain a lot of vitamins, minerals, and fiber, and they are very filling.

Let's take a look at the improvements made by the guys:

Fast-Food Freddy

Freddy's choices are limited mostly to fast food places, delivery, and take-out. Choosing the right places is important for Freddy. He needs to find fast food places that have healthy items like chicken, turkey, tuna, baked potatoes (instead of fries), salads, or a salad bar. He is not keen on eating many vegetables, but he will order a small salad if it is on the menu. Freddy found an acceptable dinner at Taco Bell. He is quite satisfied with two Soft Chicken Tacos with an order of rice. Many of his fast food choices will center on the chicken meals and not the cheeseburgers. Limiting the amount of french fries is necessary, considering the amount of calories and fat that they contain. The pizza choices will be the thin crust slices with vegetables, and not dripping with cheese. With a little planning, fast food doesn't have to be totally unhealthy.

Snack-Happy Steve

Steve's dinner options are limited by what Sally, his wife, prepares for the family. She won't be altering the family's menu, which is currently fairly healthy. Steve is going to make every effort not to continually mention that he is trying to lose a few pounds and would rather that his wife continue to prepare the meals the way she always has. This diet is designed in such a way that the people around you shouldn't be aware that you are changing anything. We are not looking for any attention or outside support. It's great if we get it, but we certainly aren't going to count on it or need it. Let's not make a big deal out of this. We are going to be eating every day for the rest of our lives. So let's get on with the business of creating a personal eating plan without the drama.

Most of Steve's improvements are going to come from avoiding second helpings, consuming less butter, and selecting healthier choices of salad dressing. Other important improvements can be made with dessert. He can also start having adult types of desserts like sherbets, frozen low-fat yogurt, or reduced calorie fudge pops, and less ice cream that is meant for the kids (The kids should be eating less ice cream too, but that's another story).

For Steve's healthy selection, he is going to have one serving of roasted chicken with long grain rice. He will also have less butter, low-cal Italian dressing with an extra large salad, and a helping of green beans.

Duck-Hook Harry

Harry is going to have to be very careful because he dines out almost every night. He is going to have to communicate with the waiters to be certain that his meals are indeed healthy. *Warning*—you cannot assume that any meal from a restaurant is healthy, no matter what the dish is called. For example, a dish like pasta primavera can be cooked in water or oil. Many other dishes can be cooked in butter or olive oil. You just don't know until you ask. Many meals from restaurants can easily add up to two thousand calories and two days worth of saturated fat. Be especially careful of Chinese restaurants that many assume are healthy. Many Chinese dishes can be extremely high in total fat, saturated fat, and sodium. Ignorance is not an excuse. The lesson is, do your homework. Harry needs to start researching the restaurants that he frequents with the same resolve that he puts into his work as an attorney. Most restaurants now have Web sites that you can browse for healthy menu choices. Recall that the USDA Web site has a link to CalorieKing.com that lists the meals from many restaurants as well as thousands of brand name foods.

Harry has done his homework choosing his improved dinner. The waiter assured him that the salmon is fresh and broiled and topped with a lemon sauce, totaling less than five hundred calories. Like Steve, he is cutting back on his intake of butter that flavors his potatoes and steamed broccoli. The meal is complemented with one five-ounce glass of Pinot Blanc.

STEP #2

Now is the time to choose a not-so-healthy dinner for the occasional time that you feel like indulging. For many, this not-so-healthy selection will be enjoyed on Saturday night or for a traditional family dinner on Sunday.

Don't be taken by surprise if you get hit with a rebellious urge to eat whatever you want, whenever you damn well please. This is not the end of the world or the end of your healthy eating habits. This is just you reasserting that you are the boss and you will not be manipulated by some stupid diet plan. Not to worry. Before you finish the meal you will probably realize that no one is telling you what to eat. This is your diet and you are making improvements because you want to. It's going to take some time to realize that you have nothing to rebel against. It's just you wanting to get healthier.

Here's what Fred, Steve, and Harry chose for their not-so-healthy dinners:

Fast-Food Freddy

Freddy is not ready to give up his Deep Dish pizza and breadsticks. He still insists that a Diet Coke is needed to wash it down. He is getting more confident that one or two not-so-healthy dinners a week is all that he will need to stay the course.

Snack-Happy Steve

Steve will occasionally sneak a second helping of dinner or a dab or two of extra butter. He hasn't totally given up his Thousand Island dressing either.

Duck-Hook Harry

Harry lets it all hang out once a week, usually on Saturday night at one of his favorite restaurants. During this meal he doesn't want to hear or think of dieting. It fact, it's the last thing on his mind. Harry figures he can soothe all of his craving during his once-a-week feast. If this is what it takes to eat healthier for the other six days, so be it. Whatever works.

Nobody knows you better than you know yourself. Come up with a plan. It will work or it won't, that's the only criteria by which to judge.

STEP #3

Next, we are going to improve our dessert choices and/or evening snack. As always, you can browse the Gold and Silver sections of the food rankings for ideas. These choices are critical because they will determine how hungry you will feel in the morning. Many people claim that they are not hungry in the morning. The remedy for that is a redistribution of caloric intake during the day. In most cases, a big breakfast, a good lunch, and a moderate dinner/dessert will do the trick. Not going to bed stuffed will also lessen morning grogginess. It will only take a few nights of light eating to improve your appetite for breakfast.

Evenings are a good time to consider the 20-minute rule. Too often, we eat dessert never considering if we are actually hungry. Many will say, "Who cares, it tastes great." I say it will taste just as great in twenty minutes. At that point you may realize that you only needed half the amount to feel satisfied. It's a win-win situation. Or you can save the dessert for your evening snack. Most of us really don't need to have dessert immediately after dinner and then have a late evening snack. One or the other should be satisfying enough. Do you really need both? I'm just asking.

Let's check in on the guys:

Fast-Food Freddy

Freddy is getting to like his improved choice of oatmeal raisin cookies with tea, instead of Chip Ahoy cookies with milk. He is also experimenting with different brands of bran muffins, making sure that they are not unhealthy belly-bombs soaked with butter. He is getting into the habit of reading the food label of every item of food that he now eats.

Snack-Happy Steve

Steve has tried a few of his wife's low-cal fudge bars. He was pleasantly surprised. He still loves ice cream, but the fudge bars are a great find.

Duck-Hook Harry

Harry doesn't have much of a sweet tooth and was never a big dessert eater. Cheesecake is the only dessert that gets him excited. He is quite content having a cup of sherbet after dinner or another glass of wine.

STEP #4

You need to select a dessert/evening snack that you can have as your not-so-healthy selection. These indulgences often are worth their weight in gold. Many times, we have an emotional attachment to dessert foods like ice cream, cookies, pie, or cake. Too often, people try to satisfy themselves with reduced calorie or substitute items. But for some things, there are no substitutes. You need to be realistic about what foods you can substitute and what foods you can't. For some people, ice cream is ice cream. For others it's heaven on Earth. If you feel that strongly about a particular food, then you should probably have it. It's not worth having two hundred calories of a low-calorie item that you don't enjoy, instead of three hundred calories of something that you do enjoy. This is especially true for those that have four hundred calories of the low-calorie item, hoping that it will eventually satisfy them. But it often doesn't.

Let's check in on what goodies the guys still like to eat:

Fast-Food Freddy

Freddy loves his Chips Ahoy cookies with milk. Now he eats only four cookies and not the whole row.

Snack-Happy Steve

Steve will join the kids and have ice cream on the weekends.

Duck-Hook Harry

One word will keep Harry happy for the rest of the week — cheesecake.

Examples of the healthy and not-so-healthy dinners, desserts, and evening snacks of Freddy, Steve, and Harry can be found in Tables 9-1 and 9-2 (Freddy), 9-3 and 9-4 (Steve), and 9-5 and 9-6 (Harry).

Table 9 – 1: Scorecard

Name: _Freddy_ Date: _Jan 18-24, 2010_ Dieting Cycle: _1_ Week#: _3_
Type of Day: _Healthy_ Calorie Goal: _2,765_ Activity Level: _Light_

Food Item	Amount	Calories	Carbohydrate	Protein	Total Fat	Saturated Fat	Trans Fat	Cholesterol	Sodium	Fiber	Sugar	Fruit Serving	Veggie Serving
Meal: _Dinner_													
Soft chicken Taco-Taco-Bell	2 ea	400	39	28	14	5	-	73	1200	4	3	-	0
Mexican Rice-Taco-Bell	1 ea	210	23	6	10	4	-	15	740	3	1	-	-
Water	12 oz	0	0	0	0	0	0	0	11	0	0	0	0
Snack: _Evening_													
Cookie-Oatmeal Raisin	1 ea	90	15	1	4	1	-	5	50	1	7	-	-
Herbal Tea-Bengal Spice	8 oz	0	0	0	0	0	0	0	0	0	0	0	0
Total:		700	77	35	28	10	0	93	2001	8	11	0	0

Table 9 – 2: Scorecard

Name: *Freddy* Date: *Jan 18-24, 2010* Dieting Cycle: *1* Week#: *3*.
Type of Day: *Not-so-Healthy* Calorie Goal: *2,765* Activity Level: *Light*

Food Item	Amount	Calories	Carbohydrate	Protein	Total Fat	Saturated Fat	Trans Fat	Cholesterol	Sodium	Fiber	Sugar	Fruit Serving	Veggie Serving
Meal: *Dinner*													
Pizza Hut-Deep Dish	2 slice	663	82	27	25	10	-	34	1358	6	8	-	0
Breadsticks	3 ea	348	53	9	12	2	-	0	457	2	2	-	-
Diet Coke	12 oz	1	0	0	0	0	0	0	6	0	0	-	-
Snack: *Evening*													
Chips-Ahoy cookies Chocolate Chip	4 ea	240	34	2	12	4	4	0	160	2	20	-	-
Whole Milk	12 oz	220	17	12	12	7	0	37	146	0	17	-	-
Total:		1472	186	50	61	23	4	71	2127	10	47	0	0

Table 9 – 3: Scorecard

Name: _Steve_ Date: _Jan 18-24, 2010_ Dieting Cycle: _1_ Week#: _3_
Type of Day: _Healthy_ Calorie Goal: _3,049_ Activity Level: _Light_

Food Item	Amount	Calories	Carbohydrate	Protein	Total Fat	Saturated Fat	Trans Fat	Cholesterol	Sodium	Fiber	Sugar	Fruit Serving	Veggie Serving
Meal: Dinner													
Dinner Salad w/greens	2 c	16	4	2	0	0	0	0	21	2	1	0	1
Italian Dressing-reduced fat	2 tbsp	40	3	0	3	1	-	0	270	0	2	-	-
Chicken—roasted	6 oz	281	0	53	6	2	-	145	126	0	0	-	-
Long grain rice	1 c	180	40	4	0	0	0	0	0	0	0	-	-
Butter	1 tbsp	100	0	0	11	7	0	30	81	0	0	-	-
Green beans w/almonds	1 c	91	8	3	5	0	-	0	144	3	3	-	1
Snack: Evening													
Caffeine free Diet Coke	12 oz	1	0	0	0	0	0	0	6	0	0	-	-
Diet Fudge Bar	1 ea	100	23	1	0	0	0	0	5	0	12	-	-
Total:		809	78	63	25	10	0	175	653	5	18	0	2

Table 9 – 4: Scorecard

Name: *Steve* Date: *Jan 18-24, 2010* Dieting Cycle: *1* Week#: *3*.
Type of Day: *Not so Healthy* Calorie Goal: *3,049* Activity Level: *Light*

Food Item	Amount	Calories	Carbohydrate	Protein	Total Fat	Saturated Fat	Trans Fat	Cholesterol	Sodium	Fiber	Sugar	Fruit Serving	Veggie Serving
Meal:							*Dinner*						
Meatloaf – Beef & pork	3 pc	665	28	59	34	12	-	267	952	3	0	-	0
Mashed Potatoes	2 serv	300	46	4	12	3	-	0	760	4	0	-	1
Butter	1 tbsp	100	0	0	11	7	0	30	81	0	0	-	-
Peas- green frozen	1 c	125	23	8	0	0	0	0	517	9	7	-	1
Soda-cola	12 oz	154	40	0	0	0	0	0	8	0	40	-	-
Dressing-Thousand Island	3 tbsp	173	7	1	16	2	-	12	404	0	6	-	-
Snack:							*Evening*						
Mixed Green Salad	2 c	16	9	2	0	0	0	0	28	2	1	-	1
Ice Cream- cookies & cream	1 serv	270	23	5	17	10	-	105	95	0	21	-	-
Chocolate Syrup	3 tbsp	150	36	2	0	0	0	0	38	0	30	-	-
Total:		1953	212	81	90	34	0	414	2883	18	105	0	3

Table 5-3. Scorecard

Name: *Harry* Date: *Jan. 18-24, 2010* Dieting Cycle: *1* Week#: *3*
Type of Day: *Healthy* Calorie Goal: *2,482* Activity Level: *Light*

Food Item	Amount	Calories	Carbohydrate	Protein	Total Fat	Saturated Fat	Trans Fat	Cholesterol	Sodium	Fiber	Sugar	Fruit Serving	Veggie Serving
Meal: *Dinner*													
Salmon - farmed broiled/blackened	6 oz.	350	0	38	21	4	-	107	104	0	0	-	-
Sauce - lemon butter dill	2 oz.	70	14	0	0	0	0	0	420	-	-	-	-
New potatoes	1 serv	145	29	6	0	-	-	0	7	4	1	-	2
Broccoli	1 serv	20	2	1	0	0	0	0	10	1	-	-	1
Butter	1 tbsp	100	0	0	11	7	0	30	81	0	0	-	1
Wine - pinot Blanc	5 oz	120	3	0	0	0	0	-	-	-	-	-	-
Snack: *Dessert*													
Sherbert/ orange	1 serv	107	22	1	1	1	-	0	34	2	18	-	-
Total:		912	70	46	33	12	0	137	656	7	19	-	4

Table 9 – 6: Scorecard

Name: _Harry_ Date: _Jan. 18-24, 2010_ Dieting Cycle: _1_ Week#: _3_.
Type of Day: _Not so Healthy_ Calorie Goal: _2,482_ Activity Level: _Light_

Food Item	Amount	Calories	Carbohydrate	Protein	Total Fat	Saturated Fat	Trans Fat	Cholesterol	Sodium	Fiber	Sugar	Fruit Serving	Veggie Serving
Meal:						_Dinner_							
Catfish-Blackened/fried	6 oz.	390	14	31	23	6	-	138	476	1	-	-	-
Creamed Spinach	1 serv	260	11	9	20	13	-	55	740	2	2	-	1
White Rice	1 c	242	53	4	0	0	0	0	0	2	-	-	-
Butter	1 tbsp	100	0	0	11	7	-	30	81	0	0	-	-
Wine-White	10 oz.	240	10	0	0	0	0	-	-	-	-	-	-
Snack:						_Dessert_							
Cheesecake	1 slice	340	30	6	21	12	-	90	270	2	25	-	-
Total:		1572	118	50	75	38	0	313	1567	7	27	-	1

STEP #5

During this week we are still shooting for workouts of low-to-moderate intensity. We still need to guard against exercising too hard. Trying to lose weight with intense exercising is a mistake. Remember, you can't out run dietary mistakes.

STEP #6

Continue to weigh yourself twice a week on the same days and at the same time. At this point you will become more familiar with the normal fluctuations in your weight according to many factors including your hydration levels, the time of day, and the sodium content of recent meals. Weight differentials of a pound or two are common even when your eating and exercise patterns are constant.

Chapter 10:
Training Camp—Week Four

The main objective of week four is to analyze the nutritional information that we have accumulated for your healthy day of eating and your not-so-healthy day of eating. These two days will give you a fairly accurate account of your current diet. Chances are good that your typical day of eating will fall somewhere between the totals of these two days. Some days may not be as good as your healthy day and some days may be better than your not-so-healthy day. More importantly, each day is probably going to be different from the next. It doesn't matter that each day will be different because you will have a detailed analysis of two days that you will be able to use to evaluate each subsequent day of eating.

STEP #1

Now we are going to copy the totals from each individual scorecard to the form titled Scorecard—Totals for the Day (appendix C). You will complete two forms, one scorecard for your healthy day of eating and another for your not-so-healthy day. Then you will add the totals of the three individual scorecards on the line indicated. The next row down from the "Total" line is for your individual goals for each of the twelve nutritional categories. Your individual goals were filled in during week one. If you haven't done so, you can refer back to step #2 of the chapter titled Play Ball!

Examples of the completed Scorecard—Totals for the Day of Freddy, Steve, and Harry for a complete day of healthy food choices and not-so-healthy food choices can be found in Tables 10-1 and 10-2 (Freddy), 10-3 and 10-4 (Steve), and 10-5 and 10-6 (Harry).

Name: *Freddy* Date: *Jan.25-31, 2010* Dieting Cycle: *1* Week#: *4*.
Type of Day: *Healthy* Calorie Goal: *2,765* Activity Level: *Light*.

Totals for the Day	Calorie	Carbohydrate	Protein	Total Fat	Saturated Fat	Trans Fat	Cholesterol	Sodium	Fiber	Sugar	Fruit Serving	Veggie Serving
Breakfast and Morning Snack	742	147	18	14	5	0	15	593	11	95	1.5	0
Lunch and Afternoon Snack	960	174	36	17	7	0	70	1417	13	55	1	2
Dinner and Dessert/Snack	700	77	35	28	10	0	93	2001	8	11	0	0
TOTAL:	2402	398	89	59	22	0	178	4,011	32	161	2.5	2
Goal:	2765	310-447	69-104	62-107	<31	0	<300	<2,300	39	<172	2-4	3-5
Score:	363 kcal. fewer	OK	OK	2 fewer	OK	OK	OK	1,711 too-many	7 too-few	OK	OK	1 serv too-few

Table 10 – 2: Scorecard

Name: _Freddy_ Date: _Jan.25-31, 2010_ Dieting Cycle: _1_ Week#: _4_ .
Type of Day: _Not so Healthy_ Calorie Goal: _2,765_ Activity Level: _Light_ .

Totals for the Day	Calorie	Carbohydrate	Protein	Total Fat	Saturated Fat	Trans Fat	Cholesterol	Sodium	Fiber	Sugar	Fruit Serving	Veggie Serving
Breakfast and Morning Snack	589	104	8	16	3	0	27	688	2	50	0	0
Lunch and Afternoon Snack	1629	179	44	86	27	10	109	1769	13	67	0	2
Dinner and Dessert/Snack	1472	186	50	61	23	4	71	2127	10	47	0	0
TOTAL:	3690	469	102	163	53	14	207	4,584	25	164	0	2
Goal:	2,765	310-447	69-104	62-107	<31	0	<300	<2,300	39	<172	2-4	3-5
Score:	928 too-many	22 g too-many	OK	56g too-many	22 g too-many	14 g Too many	OK	2,284 too-many	14 g Too few	OK	2 serv too-few	1 serv too few

Table 10 - 3. Scorecard

Name: *Steve* Date: *Jan. 25-31, 2010* Dieting Cycle: *1* Week#: *4*.
Type of Day: *Healthy* Calorie Goal: *3,049* Activity Level: *Light*.

Totals for the Day	Calorie	Carbohydrate	Protein	Total Fat	Saturated Fat	Trans Fat	Cholesterol	Sodium	Fiber	Sugar	Fruit Serving	Veggie Serving
Breakfast and Morning Snack	938	178	26	18	8	0	54	980	22	89	2	0
Lunch and Afternoon Snack	864	147	27	21	6	0	9	832	11	76	1	0
Dinner and Dessert/Snack	809	78	63	25	10	0	175	653	5	18	0	2
TOTAL:	2611	403	116	64	24	0	238	2465	38	183	3	2
Goal:	3049	338-488g	75-113g	67-117g	<33g	0	<300mg	<2300 mg	42g	<188	2-4	3-5
Score:	438 fewer	OK	2g too many	3g fewer	OK	OK	OK	165mg too many	4g too few	OK	OK	1 serv too few

Table 10 – 4: Scorecard

Name: _Steve_ Date: _Jan. 25-31, 2010_ Dieting Cycle: _1_ Week#: _4._
Type of Day: _Not so Healthy_ Calorie Goal: _3,049_ Activity Level: _Light._

Totals for the Day	Calorie	Carbohydrate	Protein	Total Fat	Saturated Fat	Trans Fat	Cholesterol	Sodium	Fiber	Sugar	Fruit Serving	Veggie Serving
Breakfast and Morning Snack	724	90	17	32	14	0	46	730	5	51	0	0
Lunch and Afternoon Snack	1014	114	47	43	20	1	127	2024	3	75	-	1
Dinner and Dessert/Snack	1953	212	81	90	34	0	414	2873	18	105	0	3
TOTAL:	3691	416	145	165	68	1	587	5637	26	231	0	4
Goal:	3,049	338-488g	75-113g	67-117g	<33g	0	<300	<2300	42g	<188	2-4	3-5
Score:	642 too many	OK	32g too-many	48g too many	35g too many	1g too many	287mg too many	3,337 too many	16g too few	43g too many	2 serv too few	OK

3. Scorecard

Name: _Harry_ Date: _Jan. 25-31, 2010_ Dieting Cycle: _1_ Week#: _4_.
Type of Day: _Healthy_ Calorie Goal: _2,482_ Activity Level: _Light_.

Totals for the Day	Calorie	Carbohydrate	Protein	Total Fat	Saturated Fat	Trans Fat	Cholesterol	Sodium	Fiber	Sugar	Fruit Serving	Veggie Serving
Breakfast and Morning Snack	709	81	24	34	8	0	20	971	9	19	0	1
Lunch and Afternoon Snack	565	77	17	22	7	0	32	1282	7	17	-	2
Dinner and Dessert/Snack	912	70	46	33	12	0	137	656	7	19	-	4
TOTAL:	2186	228	87	89	27	1	189	2909	23	55	0	7
Goal:	2482	281-406g	63-94g	56-97g	<28g	0	<300 mg	<2,300 mg	35g	<156g	2-4	3-5
Score:	296 kcal. fewer	53g fewer	OK	OK	OK	1 too many	OK	609 too many	12g too few	OK	2serv too few	2serv more

Table 10 – 6: Scorecard

Name: *Harry* Date: *Jan. 25-31, 2010* Dieting Cycle: *1* Week#: *4*.
Type of Day: *Not so Healthy* Calorie Goal: *2,482* Activity Level: *Light*.

Totals for the Day	Calorie	Carbohydrate	Protein	Total Fat	Saturated Fat	Trans Fat	Cholesterol	Sodium	Fiber	Sugar	Fruit Serving	Veggie Serving
Breakfast and Morning Snack	1297	65	51	93	29	2	693	2737	6	5	0	0
Lunch and Afternoon Snack	1008	130	28	32	14	0	172	2743	2	6	0	0
Dinner and Dessert/Snack	1572	118	50	75	38	0	313	1567	7	27	-	1
TOTAL:	3877	313	129	200	81	2	1178	7047	15	38	0	1
Goal:	2,482	281-406g	63-94g	56-97g	<28g	0	<300g	<2,300 mg	35g	<156g	2-4	3-5
Score:	1395 too-many	OK	35g too-many	103g too-many	53g too-many	2g too-many	878mg too-many	4,747 too many	20g too-few	OK	2 serv too-few	2 serv too-few

STEP #2

We are now going to look at the Scorecard—Totals for the Day for the row titled "Score." This row allows you to score your diet for the day. Two days of eating are hardly ever the same, but this does give you a good indication of the worthiness of your diet. To get your score you will compare the amounts recommended for each category versus the amounts that you actually ate. For example, if your goal for saturated fat were ≤27 grams and your total for the day added up to be 35 grams, then your score for that category would be: 8 grams too many. If your score falls within the recommended range, then you would simply write an OK in the appropriate box.

Let's check in on the guys and see how they did:

Fast-Food Freddy

Freddy's scorecard totals are listed on Tables 10-1 and 10-2. As you can see, Freddy's healthy day is not bad. In fact, it's pretty good. His only scores outside the recommended range were his sodium intake, which was 1,711 milligrams too much, and his fiber intake, which was 7 grams too few. His total fat and calorie intake were slightly outside of the recommended range and hardly worth mentioning.

Freddy's not-so-healthy day is a nightmare. One look at these totals has really opened his eyes to the dangers of blindly choosing fast foods without any restraint. He consumed too many calories, carbohydrates, total fat, saturated fat, trans fat, and sodium. He also had too little fiber, fruits, and vegetables. If Freddy ate an entire day of these foods he would gain about two pounds a week and greatly increase his risk of disease.

Snack-Happy Steve

Steve's healthy day is great. Take a look at his scorecard totals from Table 10-3. If this type of eating could be sustained, then it would only be a matter of time before Steve was back to his ideal weight. He only had four scores that were slightly outside the recommended ranges. One look at Steve's not-so-healthy day (Table 10-4) and you can see how Steve managed to gain so much weight. In total, Steve has ten scores outside the recommended ranges. The excessive amounts of total fat, saturated fat, cholesterol, and sodium are the most alarming. Just looking at the scorecard totals has been a wake-up call for Steve, who is now more motivated than ever. He never would have guessed that his not-so-healthy day was so bad.

Duck-Hook Harry

Harry's healthy day scorecard (Table 10-5) proves that you can eat out and still be healthy. But it does take some work. Generally speaking, it is incredibly easy to eat poorly and unhealthy when dining out. Just take a look at Harry's not-so-healthy day (Table 10-6), when he managed to get an astonishing ten out of twelve scores outside the recommended ranges. That is simply awful and can't happen too often. Harry is a smart guy who likes life too much to go and kill himself with his knife and fork. Harry must continue to be vigilant regarding his restaurant choices and constantly verify the content of his meals by communicating with the wait staff and selecting his restaurants according to their ability to offer healthy meals.

STEP #3

Continue to weigh yourself two times every week.

STEP #4

Continue to exercise at a low-to-moderate intensity. You may increase the frequency of your workouts (up to six times per week) but not the intensity.

Chapter 11:
Training Camp — Weeks 5 through 8

For the past four weeks, you have been primarily concerned with the improvement of your food choices (quality control). The focus for the next four weeks is going to switch to calorie restriction (quantity control). You are going to subtract five hundred calories from the calorie total that you need to maintain your weight. As I have mentioned before, calorie restriction is a major pain in the ass. Therefore, we will be applying calorie restriction for only four consecutive weeks. Keep in mind that you should not feel obligated to restrict your calories every day of the week. Some may find it helpful to restrict their calories for only five or six days per week. Remember, the goal is progress, not perfection.

This is not the time to try many new foods or exercise like a lunatic, because calorie restriction alone is enough to endure. Minor alterations or tweaking of your diet is still OK, but the main focus for the time being is going to be on the amount of calories that you consume. After four weeks of improving your diet, I'm certain that everyone is feeling much healthier and more physically fit. Chances are also good that you dropped a few pounds due to the fact that you have been exercising regularly and improving your food choices. But now we want to be certain that you continue or begin to lose the excess fat. The first four weeks of quality control have laid the foundation for weight loss by preparing you mentally and physically for the challenge of calorie restriction. The best way to do this is to closely monitor what is going into your mouth.

For the next four weeks, your goal will be to get acquainted with the amount of calories that you consume each day. Eventually, you want to be able to keep a running total of calories consumed in your head. But for now, you are going to use a pen and paper. The object of weeks five through eight is to record the calorie content of your food onto the Calorie Scorecard. A sample of the Calorie Scorecard can be found in appendix D or downloaded from http://www.rayoflife.com. You will notice that there are more columns on the Calorie Scorecard than just calories. That's because more information can be recorded if you wish. The Calorie Scorecard can also be used to obtain the exact score of your diet by calculating the percentages of your diet that are Gold, Silver, Bronze, or Zero-Value. This can be done by awarding three points for each percentage point of calories that is ranked as Gold, two points for each percentage point that is Silver, and one point for each percentage point of the diet that is Bronze. And obviously, the percent of food that is ranked as Zero-Value will be awarded zero points. Therefore, the maximum score of a diet is three hundred points (3pts x 100% Gold = 300pts).

Another feature of the Calorie Scorecard is the ability to calculate the macronutrient (carbohydrate, protein, fat) percentages of your diet. Many people have tried low-carb diets or diets that permit high amounts of fat and/or protein. This feature will allow you to calculate and see for yourself what percentages of macronutrients are best for you. Some thrive when they reduce their carbohydrate intake to around 45 percent, while others cannot function unless their percentage of carbohydrates is in the 60 percent range. Likewise, some people have fewer cravings when they consume appropriate amounts of unsaturated fat, like nuts, peanut butter, seeds, and olive oil.

This feature allows you to calculate the macronutrient percentages that are right for you. Everybody is different.

Remember, the goal is not to only eat fewer calories, but to eat fewer calories and be satisfied. This is not about testing your will power. Macronutrient content plays a vital role in achieving satiety as well as hormonal balance which stabilize cravings and blood sugar levels. Just make sure that the percentages stay within the recommended guidelines. I'm not about to tell anybody which macronutrient combination is right for them. It took me awhile to figure out what was right for me. I'm sure it will take you some time to figure out what is right for you. You may find that your macronutrient content will vary according to your activity level. Generally speaking, the need for carbohydrates will increase as your activity level increases.

You can calculate your exact diet score and/or percentage of macronutrients as you see fit. If you don't have the desire to do it, then don't. However, the calculation of calorie content is imperative. But you don't have to go crazy with this. I suggest you calculate your daily calories for five days during the first week (week five) and gradually taper off to two times a week for the duration of training camp. By then you should have a pretty good idea of the amount of calories you are consuming without having to look up many of the food items. After all, we normally eat many of the same foods during the course of a week. The goal, once again, is to be able to sit down at the end of the day and recall everything that you ate during the day and its caloric content. However, in the beginning it will be much easier and more accurate if you do it after every meal and snack.

Please keep in mind that most people (probably everyone) underreport the amount of calories that they eat each day. These errors can stem from forgetfulness, selective memory loss, improper measuring of food items, or hidden calories of many recipes due to cooking methods. If you are like most people, you can be almost certain that your calculations will be 200 to 500 calories below what you actually ate.

Also keep in mind that weight loss is a tedious and methodical process. Experts agree that the weight loss goal for an overweight person is a maximum of two pounds per week. If you do the math, two pounds of fat loss comes out to about five ounces of fat loss per day. That is the weight of a major league baseball (5.25 oz.). So the most you can lose is seven baseballs a week for a loss of two pounds. Weight loss of one pound per week is the equivalent of eight tennis balls of two ounces each. Therefore, if you need to lose thirty pounds, keep in mind that you need to lose eight dozen baseballs or 240 tennis balls, one ball at a time. For you golfers out there, thirty pounds of fat is equal to twenty-five dozen golf balls (1.62 oz. each). Hopefully these images will help you with the task at hand. Recall the marathon coach who stated that you don't run twenty-six miles but rather one mile twenty-six times. Similarly, for those losing weight, you don't lose thirty pounds but rather five ounces ninety-six times, one day at a time. You may want to gather a bucket of balls as a visual representation of the fat you wish to lose. You can then start removing balls from the bucket as you continue to lose weight. You also have to place them back in the bucket if you gain weight.

The goal is to lose between one and two pounds of fat per week. One pound of fat can be lost by eating five hundred fewer calories per day than the calories needed to maintain your weight. The reduction of five hundred calories per day would equal three thousand five hundred calories for the week which is the equivalent of one pound. Reducing your caloric intake more than five hundred calories per day is not advisable; for most people this will cause feelings of deprivation, which often leads to rebelling, complaining, and ultimately quitting. However, a small percentage of people do just fine reducing their calories by seven hundred and fifty calories a day. I don't recommend it for most people, but you can give it a try if you feel that you can handle it. Once again, these are the decisions that only you can make.

Additional weight loss can be accomplished by increasing the amount of exercise above the amount calculated during the first week of training camp. To lose one pound of fat you would need to exercise five hour per week at an intensity that would burn seven hundred calories per hour. But beware; this amount of exercise may be too much to endure. It all depends on the individual. There is a fine line between doing too much and too little. Once again, only you can decide. Keep at it until you find the proper balance for you.

Please note: Your caloric needs are going to fluctuate when you increase your activity level (e.g., from light to moderate). I suggest that you keep using the original scorecard calculations from week one. Do not change the activity level on your scorecard or recalculate your caloric needs. The only thing you are going to do is subtract the five hundred calories from the calories needed to maintain your weight. Subtracting the five hundred calories and increasing the amount of exercise will allow for weight loss between one and two pounds per week.

I am trying to minimize the paperwork as much as I can. I also don't want you to obsess about the calculations. Remember, the scale is going to be the ultimate judge as to your precise caloric needs. If you are not losing weight, you are eating too much, exercising too little, or both—regardless of calculations. The calculations are a good starting point, but the scale is the final judge.

Another option to evaluate your caloric needs would be to log back on to http://fnic.nal.usda.gov/ and follow the instruction that you were given to you in step #1 of chapter seven. But this time you would input your current information including your weight, activity level, and that you wish to lose weight. (Note that this Web site is set for weight loss at a rate of only one pound per week.)

STEP #1

Now is the time to grab a Calorie Scorecard and calculate the number of calories that you are eating for the day. A Calorie Scorecard can be found in appendix D, and is used to calculate the total calories for the day, the percentages of macronutrients in your diet, and to obtain a numerical score. Remember, your calorie goal for weeks five through eight is to eat five hundred fewer calories than the amount needed to maintain your weight. In other words, five hundred calories less than the calorie calculations you made for weeks one through four.

Let's see how the guys are doing:

<u>Fast-Food Freddy</u>

Freddy is going to record the amount of calories for the day and is interested in the percentage of macronutrients in his diet. Many of his friends are on various low carb or high protein type diets. He wants to figure out for himself the proper amount of carbohydrates that is right for him. The recommended amount of carbohydrates is between 45 percent and 65 percent. He is confused because many people are suggesting that he eats a low carb diet, but at the same time he is aware that 99 percent of all athletes eat a diet high in carbohydrates. He will vary his diet from time to time and calculate the percentages of macronutrients to see for himself what feels right. He will judge the difference between a moderate and a high carbohydrate diet according to his energy level and his ability to lose weight.

Freddy did the calculations for a typical day of eating that is listed in Table 11-1. As you can see, he consumed 2,351 calories, which was 104 percent of his 2,265 calorie goal. The

2,265 calorie goal was determined by reducing his maintenance goal of 2,765 calories by 500 calories. On this day, Freddy missed his calorie goal by 96 calories. Not bad. As a general guideline, the goal for the % Daily Calories should be between 90 and 100 percent. A % Daily Calorie score of 100 percent would mean that you eat exactly 500 calories less than the calories needed to maintain your weight. This would equate to one pound of weight loss for the week.

Also notice that his percentage of macronutrient content came out to be 58 percent carbohydrates, 15 percent protein, and 28 percent fat. These are all within the recommended guidelines.

Snack-Happy Steve

Snack-Happy Steve did a great job restricting calories. His goal was 2,549 calories (the 3,049 calories that he would need to maintain his weight minus the 500 calories required for weight loss) and he ended up having only 2,313 calories, which is 91 percent of his goal. Steve also wanted to calculate the exact score of his diet. His Calorie Scorecard (Table 11-2) represents a fairly typical day of eating for Steve. Steve's Calorie Scorecard indicates the exact score of his diet, which is 208 points. As you can see, Steve filled in the total calories for each item in the column for Calories and again in the appropriate ranking of Gold, Silver, Bronze, or Zero-Value. The calorie totals for each ranking are then divided by the overall total number of calories which gives you the proper percentages for each ranking. These percentages are then multiplied by the appropriate point value for each category, and then added, to get your exact score. Keep in mind that this score does not factor in the quantity of the diet. In other words, you can have a good quality score and still be eating too many calories.

He could improve on this score by slowly replacing his Zero-Value choices with something healthier. In this example, he scored zero points for 10 percent of his diet. But all in all, it's a great start for Steve.

Duck-Hook Harry

Good ole Harry couldn't care less about the macronutrient content of his meals or the exact score. He will focus entirely on the calorie content for the day. Judging from his Calorie Scorecard (Table 11-3), we can see that Harry is doing pretty well. Recently he has gotten into the habit of having a protein smoothie immediately after his lunchtime workout at the health club. He never thought in a million years that having a shake would be enough to satisfy him for the rest of the work day. He even gets to enjoy an oatmeal cookie and a cup of coffee before heading back to the office. As you can see, his calorie total for the day is 92 percent of his goal. Way to go Harry! At this rate he'll be losing more than one pound of fat a week.

Table 11 – 1: Scorecard

Name: _Freddy_ Date: _Feb. 1-28_ Dieting Cycle: _1_ Week#: _5-8_
Calorie Goal: _2,265_ Activity Level: _Light_.

FOOD ITEM	Amount	Meal	Calories	GOLD	SILVER	BRONZE	0 - Value	CARB	PRO	FAT
Waffles - Go-Lean	2 ea	BK	170					33	8	3
Butter	1 tsp	BK	33					1	0	6
Maple Syrup	1 oz	BK	104					27	0	0
Clif Bar -Almond	1 ea	SN	231					38	10	5
Diet Coke	12oz	SN	1					0	0	0
Chicken Sandwich/grilled	1 ea	LN	300					36	24	7
Baked Potato	1 ea	LN	310					72	7	0
Butter	1pkt	LN	33					1	0	6
Salsa	1pkt	LN	30					6	1	0
Water	12oz	LN	0					0	0	0
Trail Mix	.5 c	SN	347					34	10	22
Diet Coke	12oz	SN	1					0	0	0
PizzaHut-deep dish	2slice	DN	663					82	27	25
Beer	12oz	DN	128					11	1	0
Total Calories			2351							
% Daily Calories = (total ÷ goal) x 100			104%							
Total Calories of Gold, Silver, Bronze, 0-Value										
% Gold,Silver,Bronze= e.g. (gold ÷ total) x 100										
Points=each % Gold-3pts/Silver-2pts/Bronze-1pt										
Total Points										
Total grams of macronutrients								341g	88g	74g
Calories = each gram of CARB = 4 kcal / PRO = 4 kcal / FAT = 9 kcal								1364	352	666
% of macronutrients = e.g. (total CARB calories ÷ total calories) x 100								58%	15%	28%

Table 11 – 2: Scorecard

Name: _Steve_ Date: _Feb. 1-28_ Dieting Cycle: _1_ Week#: _5-8_
Calorie Goal: _2,549_ Activity Level: _Light_.

FOOD ITEM	Amount	Meal	Calories	GOLD	SILVER	BRONZE	0 - Value	CARB	PRO	FAT
Raisin Bran	2 c	BK	380		380					
2% Milk	1 c	BK	122		122					
Banana	1 ea	BK	105	105						
Coffee	2 c	BK	5				5			
Cream	2 oz	BK	78				78			
Yogurt/fruit	8 oz	SN	231		231					
Grape Nuts	2tbsp	SN	52		52					
PB&J sandwich	1 ea	LN	398	398						
Apple	1 ea	LN	72	72						
Diet Coke	12oz	LN	1				1			
Cup Cake	1 ea	SN	103				103			
Coffee w/cream	8 oz	SN	40				40			
Meatloaf w/gravy	6 oz	DN	420		420					
Mashed Potatoes	1serv	DN	150	150						
Dinner Salad w/greens	2 c	DN	16	16						
Italian Dressing- reduced fat	2tbsp	DN	40		40					
Diet Fudge Bar	1 ea	SN	100			100				
Total Calories			2313							
% Daily Calories = (total ÷ goal) x 100			91%							
Total Calories of Gold, Silver, Bronze, 0-Value				741	1245	100	227			
% Gold,Silver,Bronze= e.g. (gold ÷ total) x 100				32%	54%	4%	10%			
Points=each % Gold-3pts/Silver- 2pts/Bronze-1pt				96	108	4	0			
Total Points					208 *points*					
Total grams of macronutrients										
Calories = each gram of CARB = 4 kcal / PRO = 4 kcal / FAT = 9 kcal										
% of macronutrients = e.g. (total CARB calories ÷ total calories) x 100										

Table 11 – 3: Scorecard

Name: *Harry* Date: *Feb. 1-28* Dieting Cycle: *1* Week#: *5-8*.
Calorie Goal: *1,982* Activity Level: *Light*.

FOOD ITEM	Amount	Meal	Calories	GOLD	SILVER	BRONZE	0 - Value	CARB	PRO	FAT
Egg White omelet w/veggies	1serv	BK	93							
Olive Oil- cooking	1tbsp	BK	119							
Hash Browns	1serv	BK	100							
Rye Bread	1slice	BK	80							
Butter	1 tsp	BK	33							
Coffee	8oz	BK	2							
Myoplex protein shake	16oz	LN	450							
Oatmeal cookie	2 ea	LN	180							
Coffee	8oz	LN	2							
Turkey Breast w/o skin	6oz	DN	200							
Sweet Potato	1 ea	DN	110							
Green beans w/almonds	1serv	DN	91							
Salad/tomato/croutons	2 c	DN	69							
Dressing-balsamic	2tbsp	DN	80							
Butter	1tbsp	DN	100							
Wine	5oz	DN	120							
Total Calories			1829							
% Daily Calories = (total ÷ goal) x 100			92%							
Total Calories of Gold, Silver, Bronze, 0-Value										
% Gold,Silver,Bronze= e.g. (gold ÷ total) x 100										
Points=each % Gold-3pts/Silver-2pts/Bronze-1pt										
Total Points										
Total grams of macronutrients										
Calories = each gram of CARB = 4 kcal / PRO = 4 kcal / FAT = 9 kcal										
% of macronutrients = e.g. (total CARB calories ÷ total calories) x 100										

STEP #2

Continue to weigh yourself religiously twice a week. You'll be learning a lot about yourself and what it takes to lose weight as the weeks go by. By now, weighing yourself should become less emotionally charged. Remember that you're in this for the long haul. You can't be on pins and needles every time that you step on the scale. Having that attitude is a sure way to burn out. The desire to lose weight can't be continuously on the front burner. It needs to be on the back burner simmering away, unnoticed, as you carry on with your life. Deep inside, you know that you want to be fit. That desire to lose the weight is all you need to succeed. Your desire is nobody else's business. Just keep at it, methodically and quietly at your own pace.

STEP #3

Continue to exercise regularly. For this portion of training camp your exercise should remain at low-to-moderate intensity. We are still in phase one of our exercise routine. If you are ready, feel free to increase the number of times that you exercise per week, and/or the duration of those workouts. The additional exercise will aid in the weight loss process. However, this is not the time to increase the intensity. Your exercise should be giving you more energy during the day and not leaving you exhausted. Remember that intense workouts will make it increasingly more difficult to control your eating. There will be plenty of time to work out intensely, just not now.

Please note: You may continue with calorie restriction for another week or two if you desire. Recall that you have four wild-card weeks to use during the course of a year.

Chapter 12:
The Season—Weeks 9 through 12

Now is the time for your diet to go on automatic pilot. You will no longer be restricting calories or filling out scorecards. This is when you will be able to determine just how much you have improved your diet. How well do you eat without the continued focus on food? And more importantly, how much of the motivation, that is common at the start of a dieting program, do you manage to keep? During training camp, you practiced various dieting skills and methodically improved your diet one meal at a time. Now is the time to maintain your weight and to make the dietary improvements a normal part of your life.

STEP #1

The most important thing during the season is to continue the habit of weighing yourself twice a week. After eight weeks of effort, it is easy to go back to old familiar habits. The scale is the only means available to keep you honest. It is fairly easy to kid yourself into thinking that you are eating well enough to maintain your weight. This is no time to think; this is a time to know. The scale will take all the thinking out of the equation. The scale deals with facts; you gained weight, lost weight, or stayed the same. The rest is nonsense. So keep hopping on that scale.

STEP #2

It's time to make changes to your exercise routine. Exercise during the season will be shifting into phase two. As you recall, in phase one (weeks one through eight) our intention was to exercise at low-to-moderate intensity. During phase two you will turn up the intensity of your workouts as the focus on food shifts to the back burner. This is a great way to stay fresh and motivated throughout the entire year. Remember, *Diet for the Sports-Minded Male* advocates that exercise and dieting have an inverse relationship: when the focus on one becomes more intense, the focus on the other declines. In other words, the importance of your food choices and the restriction of calories have been front and center for the last eight weeks, while your exercise routine complemented the process. It is now time for exercise to take a more prominent role as your food choices complement your training. The goal is to increase the amount of exercise to five hours per week (if you haven't already). The increase in the amount of exercise will be extremely helpful in maintaining the weight loss that was achieved during training camp.

Let's see how the guys are handling the transition from training camp to the season:

Fast-Food Freddy

Freddy has gotten comfortable going to the gym on a regular basis and exercising with his girlfriend on the weekends. His cardiovascular system and muscles have adapted well during the last two months and he is now ready to take it to the next level. Freddy's phase one workouts have been up-tempo, moderate weight, circuit training type routines. He will now switch to the more traditional routine of eight to twelve repetitions of progressive overload. During his progressive overload training he will intentionally challenge himself with more weight (resistance) until the new weight becomes manageable (completing 8-12 reps). Once the body adapts to the new weight he will immediately challenge the body by overloading it with additional weight, performing more sets or repetitions, or reducing his recovery time. The new focus on exercise will help Freddy maintain the many gains that he made during training camp. You are trying to create a cycle of having your motivation continually flow from diet to exercise, without ever getting stale. One hand washes the other: improvements due to dieting will create the inspiration for exercise, and vice versa. This cycle can be maintained as long as you honor the inverse relationship between diet and exercise.

Snack-Happy Steve

Steve's walking/jogging routine is going well. He has increased his mileage and is now jogging about half of the time that he's out on the road. During phase two he will be increasing the intensity a bit by adding some hills to his jogging route. He will begin by walking the hills then gradually jogging small portions. Steve did manage to get his stationary bike fixed, which will come in handy on raining days and reduce the stress to his big body. He regularly shoots baskets with his boys after school and/or after dinner. He made a promise to himself that he will be able to play one-on-one with his boys when they are seniors in high school. That's a great motivational goal for the next few years.

Duck-Hook Harry

Harry now exercises between three and five days a week at the health club and plays golf at least once a week. He walks on the treadmill during lunch with headphones tuned in to the many televisions flickering away. During his walk, he catches up on the news and his stocks, and then proceeds to the steam room. A quick stop at the club café for a smoothie, and then back to work. Harry has also tried a few yoga classes. You have to admire Harry's willingness to try new things. However, he is still working up the courage to start a weight lifting program with the help of a trainer. Not a bad idea. He has never touched a weight in his life, and he is no longer a spring chicken.

Chapter 13:
Off-Season — Weeks 13 through 16

First of all, we need to combat the ridiculous notion that going off your diet is somehow considered a failure. Since when are we supposed to be perfect? The greatest athletes in the world have an off-season, so why can't we? This diet is designed for the purpose of getting healthy and fit, and remaining that way. The best way for that *not* to happen is to try to be perfect for the rest of your life. I'll say it again: there's a time to lose, a time to gain, and a time to stay the same. That's life; we are not going to fight it. It is only natural that you may feel like loosening up a bit after twelve weeks of disciplined action. However, do not look at this off-season as a license to pig out.

The goal during the off-season is to regain no more than 25 percent of the weight lost. What we are looking for is a four-step–forward, one-step-back scenario. After three dieting cycles (one year), you are looking at a net gain of nine steps forward. And that's just the first year. The goal is for your weight to fluctuate only two or three pounds from your ideal weight, for the rest of your life.

Exercise during the off-season is going to be vital. Five hours per week is recommended to prevent or limit the regaining of weight. Continuing to weigh yourself twice a week is also vital. The last thing you want to do is wake up one day to find that you have gained seven pounds. Don't make the mistake of thinking that your pants still fit the same. Pants do stretch. Boy, can they stretch. Guys are also real good at sneaking that belly over their belts. It's going to be a lot more difficult to continue to overeat, if you are weighing yourself twice every week. If you find that you are forgetting to weigh yourself, you will probably find that you have gained weight. You can almost count on it. Anyway, that's been my experience.

STEP #1

Continue to weigh yourself two times every week (have I mentioned that already?). This is never as important as it is now. In fact, if you do nothing else that I have suggested, at least continue to weigh yourself twice a week for the rest of your life. My theory is that no one can consciously watch themselves become fat, week after week, pound after pound. I don't know anyone who watched the numbers on the scale continue to climb week after week. The only way to get fat is to ignore your weight for an extended period of time, and then one day, out of the blue, you find yourself ten pounds fatter. Sound familiar? Hopefully not, but it does happen.

STEP #2

During the off-season your main focus will switch from food to exercise. For the past three months you have been exercising primarily at a low-to-moderate intensity. But now is the time when you can let it all hang out and exercise as much and as hard as you like. The timing is perfect for two reasons. One reason is that you are now physiologically ready for more intense workouts. You have been cautiously preparing your cardiovascular system for the past twelve weeks. Second, your motivation level for dieting is probably starting to wane and can now be renewed by channeling it into your exercise routine. Alternating the focus from food to exercise allows you to stay motivated all year long.

Let's see what the guys are doing:

Fast-Food Freddy

Freddy is now mentally and physiologically ready to take his workouts to the next level. He will now begin to work out as hard as he wishes and really begin to see major changes in his body. Some of the extra calories that he will consume during the off-season have a good chance of being burned off during his prolonged and intense training sessions. It is difficult to outrun all dietary indiscretions, but he is going to try.

Snack-Happy Steve

Steve is progressing slowly and safely toward his goal of running a 10-K without having to walk. During this off-season Steve has no intention of regaining any of the weight that he has lost. Steve is also going to address his lack of flexibility at this time. He has noticed that he is stiffer than ever after his workouts. He is not sure if it's because he is getting older or he has been inactive for so long. In either case, he needs to do something. He has elected to try his wife's DVD called *Power Yoga for Beginners* with Rodney Yee. He refuses to take a yoga class in public, but is willing to try a few DVD's in the privacy of his own home.

Duck-Hook Harry

Harry has decided to start resistance training during this off-season. Harry can now put all his energy into this new endeavor and give his mind a rest from the constant focus on food. He will begin his training sessions with the help of a personal trainer to ensure that his program is fundamentally sound, effective, and safe.

STEP #3

For the past few months you have been on the offensive trying hard to improve your diet and restrict your caloric intake. Now is the time to play dee-fence. Feel free to loosen-up without letting go. If you are having a hard time controlling your diet and staying motivated, hang in there. Do the best that you can until your motivation returns. It always does. But until it does, you need to play some defense. Overeating one slice of pizza is better than overeating two slices of pizza. Eating right shouldn't be an all or nothing proposition. Try not to limit yourself to a *pig-or-perfect* mentality. There is plenty of gray area in between. Staying in that gray area is going to save you. Don't dig yourself into such a big hole that you can't climb back out. Hang in there the best you can until your motivation returns for the next training camp. Think back on all that you have accomplished. Gaining a few pounds is all part of the master plan. But having a total collapse of self control can't happen. Always remember that defense wins games.

You'll begin to realize that the off-season is the most important season of them all. Many find this time more challenging than training camp or the season. Remember one of the golden rules: It's more important not to have a really bad eating day than it is to have a really good eating day. Just do the math. On a good eating day you may eat five hundred less calories of healthy food than you would need to maintain your weight. But on a really bad day you can easily eat two thousand extra calories of complete crap. Do you see what I mean?

Extra Points

The guidelines and recommendations that I have made in this book can all be fine-tuned to meet your individual needs. The main concepts are there to use as you see fit. If something does not make sense to you, don't do it. I'll say it for the last time: this is your diet, not mine. Don't let minor details get in the way of becoming healthier and fit. The results that you get are the only criteria to judge whether your diet is working or not. The goal is to look good, feel better, and be confident that the improvements that you make can be sustained indefinitely. How you achieve that goal is up to you. However, I do recommend that you follow my suggestions as close as you can before making major alterations.

Quite often, it comes down to balancing the extremes of trying to do too much and doing too little. If you do too much you will burn out and find a reason to quit. If you do too little you will not get the results as quickly as you would like. And results are the only things that are going to keep you motivated for the long haul. You will no longer need to rely on self-discipline once you are feeling better. Feeling better is the only motivation you will need. At that point the diet plan simply becomes your normal way of life.

I suggest that you don't worry too much in the beginning about getting huge amounts of weight loss. That will come in time. The important thing now is to start creating healthier habits that can be sustained for a lifetime. It is much more beneficial to gain confidence in a good solid diet plan than it is to bounce around from one stupid fad diet to the next. The steady improvements throughout the year will add up to much more than the occasional gains of a deprivation type diet.

Keep in mind that the first dieting cycle is the toughest. The upcoming dieting cycles should be a breeze compared to the first. After the first cycle, you will know the system and how to complete the scorecards. In the future, you will simply be filling out scorecards for different meals and snacks. For example, if you filled out a scorecard for cold cereal during your first dieting cycle, you would then fill out a scorecard for a different breakfast (e.g., oatmeal) for the second diet cycle. And you probably won't need to complete another not-so-healthy scorecard for the rest of your life. After the first cycle, you will understand quite well how easy it is to eat a not-so-healthy diet.

I would also like to mention an alternative to the typical sixteen-week cycle. This alterative is for those who are satisfied with their current diet and have already completed scorecards for all their meals and snacks. If that is case, you will begin the first four weeks of training camp with calorie restriction and not the improvement of your food choices. However, I do not recommend that you restrict calories for more than six consecutive weeks. Therefore, I recommend that you prolong your season and off-season so that the cycles remain sixteen weeks.

When making alterations, the most important thing to remember is to have a goal for each week of the year. For each week you would have one of four goals that would be equally distributed throughout the year. You would be improving your food choices (training camp-quality control), restricting calories (training camp-quantity control), maintaining your weight (season), or gaining as little weight as possible (off-season). How you construct the weeks of the year is ultimately up to you. But once again, I do recommend that you follow my suggestions before making drastic changes.

CONCLUSION

Never forget that you have what it takes to be as healthy and fit as you like. Don't get bent out of shape about the details. You'll figure it all-out in due time. Sports-minded males are one of the few groups in America that can be successful improving their diets. If you're anything like the sports-minded males that I know, you'll do just fine. You can do whatever you set your mind to. You just have to set your mind to do it. Never forget that you already know more than enough to improve your health. Don't sell yourself short. This diet stuff is not complicated. All you need to do is work the plan and have a little patience. Recall that over the years, coaches have demonstrated to us how to hit a baseball, throw a football, and shoot a basketball. But for the most part, we had to figure out how to do it all by ourselves. The same goes for dieting. You'll put in the work and you'll figure it out. Others may know more about nutrition than you, but no one should be able to outwork you. And that is what counts most. With a little coaching, sports-minded males can have a whole new and positive outlook regarding diet. With the slightest bit of creativity and a touch of patience, I truly believe that sports-minded males can get as fit as they want. I hope this book can supply the direction to keep you on the path toward health and fitness. You deserve it. Go get it!

If you have any questions or comments, I can be reached at http://www.rayoflife.com. You can also e-mail me at rayoflife@mindspring.com. Looking forward to hearing from you and good luck!

About the Author

RAY BURIGO, MS, RD, CISSN, CPT

Ray Burigo is the creator of the Ray of Life Health System (http://www.rayoflife.com) that specializes in wellness, weight loss, and sports nutrition. Ray has twenty-one years experience counseling and training clients in New York City, West Hampton Beach, NY, and currently in Los Angeles, CA.

Ray is a registered dietitian (RD) with a Master of Science in nutrition from California State University, Northridge. His graduate thesis, titled *Development of Nutritional Information for Athletes*, examined the behaviors, concerns, and nutritional knowledge of collegiate athletes for the purpose of developing educational materials.

He is certified with the International Society of Sports Nutrition (CISSN) as a sports nutritionist and by Marymount Manhattan College, NYC, as a personal trainer (CPT). Ray also received certification as a health specialist from the American Health Sciences Institute, which specializes in raw food, vegetarian, and vegan diets.

Before embarking on his second career in health, Ray spent thirteen years in sales and marketing after earning a BBA in Marketing from Iona College in New Rochelle, N.Y.

Appendices

Appendix A
Dietary Guidelines for Various Calorie Needs

(continued on next page)

Calories Per Day	CARBOHYDRATE	PROTEIN (recommended)	PROTEIN (acceptable)	TOTAL FAT	SATURATED FAT	TRANS FAT
	45% to 65%	10% to 15%	10% to 35%	20% to 35%	<10%	0 – sparingly (<1% of total kcal)
1,500	169g – 244g	38g – 56g	38g – 131g	33g – 58g	<17g	sparingly
1,750	197g – 284g	44g – 66g	44g – 153g	39g – 68g	<20g	sparingly
2,000	225g – 325g	50g – 75g	50g – 175g	44g – 78g	<22g	sparingly
2,250	253g – 366g	57g – 85g	57g – 197g	50g – 88g	<25g	sparingly
2,500	281g – 406g	63g – 94g	63g – 219g	56g – 97g	<28g	sparingly
2,750	310g – 447g	69g – 104g	69g – 241g	62g – 107g	<31g	sparingly
3,000	338g – 488g	75g – 113g	75g – 263g	67g – 117g	<33g	sparingly
3,250	366g – 528g	82g – 122g	82g – 285g	73g – 127g	<36g	sparingly
3,500	394g – 567g	88g – 131g	88g – 306g	78g – 136g	<39g	sparingly
3,750	422g – 609g	94g – 141g	94g – 328g	84g – 146g	<42g	sparingly
4,000	450g – 650g	100g – 150g	100g – 350g	89g – 155g	<44g	sparingly
4,250	478g – 691g	107g – 160g	107g – 372g	95g – 165g	<47g	sparingly
4,500	506g – 731g	113g – 169g	113g – 394g	100g – 175g	<50g	sparingly

Appendix A
Dietary Guidelines for Various Calorie Needs

Calories Per Day	CHOLESTEROL	SODIUM	FIBER	SUGAR	FRUIT SERVINGS	VEGETABLE SERVINGS
	< 300 milligrams	< 2,300 milligrams	14 grams per 1000 calories	< 25% of total calories	between 2 - 4 servings	between 3 - 5 servings
1,500	< 300 mg	< 2,300mg	21g	<94g	2-4 servings	3-5 servings
1,750	< 300 mg	< 2,300mg	25g	<109g	2-4 servings	3-5 servings
2,000	< 300 mg	< 2,300mg	28g	<125g	2-4 servings	3-5 servings
2,250	< 300 mg	< 2,300mg	32g	<141g	2-4 servings	3-5 servings
2,500	< 300 mg	< 2,300mg	35g	<156g	2-4 servings	3-5 servings
2,750	< 300 mg	< 2,300mg	39g	<172g	2-4 servings	3-5 servings
3,000	< 300 mg	< 2,300mg	42g	<188g	2-4 servings	3-5 servings
3,250	< 300 mg	< 2,300mg	46g	<204g	2-4 servings	3-5 servings
3,500	< 300 mg	< 2,300mg	49g	<219g	2-4 servings	3-5 servings
3,750	< 300 mg	< 2,300mg	53g	<235g	2-4 servings	3-5 servings
4,000	< 300 mg	< 2,300mg	56g	<250g	2-4 servings	3-5 servings
4,250	< 300 mg	< 2,300mg	60g	<266g	2-4 servings	3-5 servings
4,500	< 300 mg	< 2,300mg	63g	<281g	2-4 servings	3-5 servings

Appendix B
SCORECARD - Meal and Snack

Name: _____

Type of Day: _____

Date: _____   Dieting Cycle: _____   Calorie Goal: _____   Activity Level: _____   Week#: _____

Food Item	Amount	Calories	Carbohydrate	Protein	Total Fat	Saturated Fat	Trans Fat	Cholesterol	Sodium	Fiber	Sugar	Fruit Serving	Veggie Serving
Meal:													
Snack:													
Total:													

Appendix C

SCORECARD - Totals for the Day

Name: _____ Date: _____ Dieting Cycle: _____ Week#: _____

Type of Day: _____ Calorie Goal: _____ Activity Level: _____

Food Item	Amount	Calories	Carbohydrate	Protein	Total Fat	Saturated Fat	Trans Fat	Cholesterol	Sodium	Fiber	Sugar	Fruit Serving	Veggie Serving
Breakfast and Morning Snack													
Lunch and Afternoon Snack													
Dinner and Dessert/Snack													
Totals													
Goals:													
Score:													

Appendix D
Calorie Scorecard

Name: _____ Date: _____ Dieting Cycle: _____ Week#: _____
Type of Day: _____ Calorie Goal: _____ Activity Level: _____

FOOD ITEM	Amount	Meal	Calories	GOLD	SILVER	BRONZE	0 - Value	CARB	PRO	FAT

Total Calories										
% Daily Calories = (total ÷ goal) x 100										
Total Calories of Gold, Silver, Bronze, 0-Value										
% Gold,Silver,Bronze= e.g. (gold ÷ total) x 100										
Points=each % Gold-3pts/Silver-2pts/Bronze-1pt										
Total Points										
Total grams of macronutrients										
Calories = each gram of CARB = 4 kcal / PRO = 4 kcal / FAT = 9 kcal										
% of macronutrients = e.g. (total CARB calories ÷ total calories) x 100										

Appendix E
FOOD RANKINGS
Table of Contents

Appendix E

FOOD RANKINGS

ABBREVIATIONS

Amt - Amount
Food - Food
Brand - Brand
Kcal - Calories
CHO - Carbohydrate (grams)
PRO - Protein (grams)
FAT - Total fat (grams)
Sat Fat - Saturated fat (grams)
Trans Fat - Trans fat (grams)
Chol- Cholesterol (milligrams)
Sodium - Sodium (milligrams)
Fiber - Fiber (grams)
Sugar- Sugar (grams)
Fruit - Fruit (servings)
Veggie - Vegetables (servings)

ABBREVIATIONS OF PRODUCT AMOUNTS

c - cup
ea. - each
oz. - once
pc. - piece
pkt. - packet
serv - serving
sl - slice
tsp - teaspoon
tbsp - tablespoon

Note: USDA listed as Brand signifies a standard measurement of the USDA

Nutritional information for the Food Rankings is provided with permission from The Food Processor SQL© Nutrition Analysis Software (Version 10.1.0) from ESHA Research, Salem, Oregon.

MEAL: BREAKFAST   GROUP: 1   CATEGORY: HOT CEREAL

SELECTION TIPS: Look to see how much **fiber** and **sugar** are in the product. High fiber (>4 grams) merits a Gold ranking. Amounts of **protein** are typically greater than that of cold cereals.

Amt	Food	Brand	Kcal	CHO	PRO	FAT	Sat Fat	Trans Fat	Chol	Sodium	Fiber	Sugar	Fruit	Veggie
								GOLD						
½ c Dry	Steel Cut Oatmeal	John McCann	300	52	8	4	0	0	0	0	8	0	-	-
1 c	Whole Grain Pilaf	Kashi	340	60	12	6	0	0	0	30	12	0	-	-
								SILVER						
1 serv	Hot Cereal in a Cup	Health Valley	240	45	10	3	0	0	0	240	4	9	-	-
1 c	Hot Cereal-10 Grain	Health Valley	220	41	12	2	0	0	0	210	5	8	-	-
1 c	Hot Multi-Grain Oatmeal	Quaker Oats	143	32	5	1	0	0	0	7	5	0	-	-
								BRONZE						
1 serv	Oatmeal-cinnamon spice	Quaker Oats	170	35	4	2	0	0	0	246	3	16	-	-
1 serv	Farina- apple cinnamon	Cream of Wheat	130	29	2	0	0	0	0	160	1	16	-	-
1 serv	Oatmeal- maple & brown sugar	Quaker Oats	157	32	4	2	0	0	0	261	3	14	-	-
1 serv	Farina Original	Cream of Wheat	90	17	3	0	0	0	0	170	1	0	-	-

ZERO-VALUE - does not apply

MEAL: BREAKFAST   GROUP: 2   CATEGORY: COLD CEREAL

SELECTION TIPS: The first thing to look at is the amount of **fiber** and **sugar**. Gold ranking has >5 grams of fiber while sugar is < 7 grams. Gold and Silver products also have >3 grams of **protein**. Note: the high sugar amount for Raisin Bran is partially due to the raisins (a good thing) and not added sugar (a bad thing).

Amt	Food	Brand	Kcal	CHO	PRO	FAT	Sat Fat	Trans Fat	Chol	Sodium	Fiber	Sugar	Fruit	Veggie
						GOLD								
1 c	Go-Lean	Kashi	151	31	14	1	0	0	0	88	10	6	-	-
1 c	Cheerios	General Mills	111	22	4	2	0	0	0	210	6	0	-	-
1 serv	Shredded Wheat	Post	160	37	5	1	0	0	0	0	6	0	-	-
						SILVER								
½ c	Grape Nuts	Post	208	47	6	1	0	0	0	354	5	7	-	-
1 c	Wheaties	General Mills	107	24	3	1	0	0	0	218	3	4	-	-
1 c	Raisin Bran	Post	190	46	4	1	0	0	0	300	8	19	-	-
						BRONZE								
1 c	Special K	Kellogg's	117	22	7	0	0	0	0	224	1	4	-	-
1 c	Rice Krispies	Kellogg's	102	23	2	0	0	0	0	251	0	2	-	-
1 c	Corn Flakes	Kellogg's	101	24	2	0	0	0	0	202	1	3	-	-
						ZERO-VALUE								
1 c	Lucky Charms	General Mills	114	25	2	1	0	0	0	203	1	13	-	-
1 c	Cap N Crunch	Quaker Oats	144	31	2	2	1	0	0	270	1	16	-	-
1 c	Frosted Flakes	Kellogg's	152	37	1	0	0	0	0	198	1	16	-	-

MEAL: BREAKFAST		GROUP: 3				CATEGORY: CEREAL TOPPINGS								

SELECTION TIPS: A great way to add fruit to your diet. Be careful with the amounts of nuts and dried fruit (they both have a fair amount of **calories**). Milk products are listed under cold beverages (Group 37).

Amt	Food	Brand	Kcal	CHO	PRO	FAT	Sat Fat	Trans Fat	Chol	Sodium	Fiber	Sugar	Fruit	Veggie
						GOLD								
2 tbsp	Raisins	USDA	60	16	0.7	0	0	0	0	2.4	1	-	0.5	-
1 tbsp	Almonds, slivers	USDA	39	1.3	1.4	3.4	0.3	0	0	0	0.8	0.3	-	-
½ ea	Banana	USDA	55	15	0.5	0	0	0	0	0	1.5	9.5	0.3	-
1 tsp	Cinnamon	USDA	6	1.8	0	0	0	0	0	0.6	1.3	0	-	-
20 ea	Blueberries	USDA	16	4	0	0	0	0	0	0	1	3	0.2	-
½ c	Strawberries	USDA	27	6	0.5	0	0	0	0	0.8	1.7	4	0.5	-
1 tbsp	Flax Seed, ground	USDA	40	2	1.5	3	0	0	0	0	1.5	0	-	-
						SILVER - does not apply								
						BRONZE								
1 tbsp	Brown Sugar	USDA	45	12	0	0	0	0	0	0	0	12	-	-
1 tbsp	Maple Syrup	USDA	52	13	0	0	0	0	0	1.8	0	12	-	-
1 tbsp	Honey	USDA	63	18	0	0	0	0	0	0	0	15	-	-
						ZERO-VALUE - does not apply								

MEAL: BREAKFAST GROUP: 4 CATEGORY: BREADS

SELECTION TIPS: The easiest way to pick healthy bread is to look at the **fiber** content (3-4 grams per serving is good). Also look for the words "whole wheat" or "whole grain" or "100% whole wheat flour" listed first on the ingredients list.

Amt	Food	Brand	Kcal	CHO	PRO	FAT	Sat Fat	Trans Fat	Chol	Sodium	Fiber	Sugar	Fruit	Veggie
							GOLD							
1 pc.	Whole Grain bread	Natural Ovens	60	14	2	1	0	0	0	80	5	1	-	-
1 ea	Multi-Grain English Muffin	Oroweat	150	32	5	2	0	0	0	170	4	4	-	-
1 ea	Bagel-whole Wheat	Natural Ovens	170	37	6	2	0	0	0	200	6	4	-	-
							SILVER							
1 pc.	Bread-Pumpernickel	Pepperidge Farm	80	15	3	1	0	0	0	230	2	1	-	-
1 pc.	Bread-Whole Wheat	Oroweat	70	14	3	1	0	0	0	160	2	2	-	-
1 pc.	Bread, 7-grain	USDA	65	12	2.6	1	0	0	0	127	1.6	2.6	-	-
							BRONZE							
1 pc.	White Bread	Oroweat	110	20	3	2	0	0	0	240	1	4	-	-
1 pc.	Bread-Cinnamon Swirl	Pepperidge Farm	80	14	3	2	0	0	0	105	1	6	-	-
1 ea	Bagel-plain	Thomas'	290	56	11	2	0	0	0	540	3	7	-	-

ZERO-VALUE - does not apply

MEAL: BREAKFAST   GROUP: 5   CATEGORY: BREAD TOPPINGS

SELECTION TIPS: Watch for the **fat** content in butter, margarine, and cheese spreads. Peanut butter is high in fat, but it's the good fat. Look for margarines that do not contain **trans fats** or the word "hydrogenated" within the ingredients.

Amt	Food	Brand	Kcal	CHO	PRO	FAT	Sat Fat	Trans Fat	Chol	Sodium	Fiber	Sugar	Fruit	Veggie
						GOLD								
1 tbsp	100% Fruit Spread	Smucker's	40	10	0	0	0	0	0	0	0	8	-	-
1 tbsp	Peanut Butter	Smucker's	100	4	4	8	1	0	0	0	1	1	-	-
1 tbsp	Almond Butter	USDA	85	3	4	8	1	0	0	0	2	0	-	-
						SILVER								
1 tbsp	Jam, Strawberry	USDA	50	13	0	0	0	0	0	0	0	12	-	-
1 tbsp	Jelly, Grape	USDA	50	13	0	0	0	0	0	0	0	12	-	-
1 tbsp	Cream Cheese, fat free	Philadelphia	40	10	0	0	0	0	0	0	0	8	-	-
						BRONZE								
1 tbsp	Cream Cheese, light	Philadelphia	35	1	1.5	2.5	1.8	-	7.5	75	0	1	-	-
1 serv	Cream Cheese, whipped	USDA	35	0	1	3	2	0	11	30	1	0	-	-
1 serv	Cream Cheese	USDA	50	0.4	1.1	5.1	3.2	-	16	43	0	0	-	-
1 tbs	Cream Cheese, substitute	Tofutti Brands	80	1	1	8	2	-	0	135	0	0	-	-
						ZERO-VALUE								
1 tbsp	Butter	USDA	100	0	0	11	7	-	30	81	0	0	-	-
1 tbsp	Margarine	Land o Lakes	100	0	0	11	2	2	0	105	0	0	-	-

MEAL: BREAKFAST   GROUP: 6   CATEGORY: EGG DISHES

SELECTION TIPS: Experts are now saying that one whole egg per day is O.K. The rest should be egg whites. The yolk of the egg contains all the **cholesterol** but also contains many important nutrients. Limit the amount of products containing high amounts of **saturated fat** like bacon, sausage, and cheese.

Amt	Food	Brand	Kcal	CHO	PRO	FAT	Sat Fat	Trans Fat	Chol	Sodium	Fiber	Sugar	Fruit	Veggie
							GOLD							
1 ea	Egg White, cooked	USDA	17	0	4	0	0	0	0	55	0	0	-	-
1 serv	Egg White Omelet, onions & peppers	USDA	93	6.4	15	0.3	0	0	0	225	1.3	3.5	-	0.5
							SILVER							
1 ea	Egg, hard boiled	USDA	78	1	6	5	2	-	212	62	0	1	-	-
1 ea	Omelet, veggies, 1 egg	USDA	110	2	8	8	2	-	223	108	1	1	-	0.4
1 ea	Egg, fried in veg. oil	USDA	121	0	6	11	2	-	196	97	0	0	-	-
							BRONZE							
1 ea	French Toast w/sausage	USDA	432	34	22	23	7	-	251	1068	1	0	-	-
1 ea	Scrambled eggs, ham & cheese	USDA	156	2	11	11	4	-	198	372	0	0	-	-
1 ea	Omelet, sausage	USDA	167	2	11	13	4	-	267	294	0	2	-	-

ZERO-VALUE - does not apply

MEAL: BREAKFAST   GROUP: 7   CATEGORY: SIDE ORDERS

SELECTION TIPS: Be careful! Products with the same names can have different nutritional content. You got to read the labels, especially the serving sizes. One company's serving size may be twice that of another company. Check out the **fat** and **saturated** fat content before eating.

Amt	Food	Brand	Kcal	CHO	PRO	FAT	Sat Fat	Trans Fat	Chol	Sodium	Fiber	Sugar	Fruit	Veggie
						GOLD								
1 serv	Fruit Cup	USDA	90	22	1	0	0	0	0	10	1	19	0.5	-
1 serv	Grits, corn	Quaker Oats	96	22	2.4	0.3	0.03	-	0	304	1.3	0.08	-	-
½ c	Black Beans	USDA	113	20	7.6	0.5	0.1	0	0	0.9	7.5	-	-	-
						SILVER								
1 serv	Home Fries	USDA	120	22	2	3	1.5	-	0	20	2	0	-	-
1 serv	Vegetable Meat Sausage	USDA	70	5	8	3	0.5	0	0	330	2	2	-	-
1 ea	Canadian Bacon	USDA	68	1	9.5	2.7	1	-	27	568	-	0.8	-	-
						BRONZE								
1 serv	Sausage, pork	USDA	82	0	3.9	7.3	2.6	-	19	200	0	0.2	-	-
1 ea	Sausage, turkey	USDA	65	0	6.2	4.7	1.6	-	23	191	0	0	-	-
1 ea	Bacon, fried	USDA	42	0.1	3	3.2	1.1	0	8.9	192	0	0	-	-
1 serv	Hash Browns	USDA	136	13	1.8	9.2	1.6	-	0	289	1.7	0.06	-	-

ZERO-VALUE - does not apply

MEAL: BREAKFAST		GROUP: 8							CATEGORY: FRUIT/DAIRY				

SELECTION TIPS: The sugar content on the label usually applies to "added sugar." But that is not the case with fruit and dairy products. Do not be alarmed because of the high sugar content. The sugars in fruit and dairy products are natural sugars and not the empty **calories** that are added to soda, pastries, candy, and other inferior foods. Look for non-fat or low-fat products to limit the amount of **fat** and **saturated fat**. **Sodium** is often high in some cottage cheeses.

Amt	Food	Brand	Kcal	CHO	PRO	FAT	Sat Fat	Trans Fat	Chol	Sodium	Fiber	Sugar	Fruit	Veggie
								GOLD						
1 serv	Yogurt, non-fat	Nancy's	120	17	12	0	0	0	5	180	0	17	-	-
1 ea	Banana, medium	USDA	105	27	1	0	0	0	0	1	3	14	1	-
1 c	Strawberry	USDA	53	13	1	0	0	0	0	1.6	3.3	8	1	-
1 c	Pineapple, diced	USDA	74	20	1	0	0	0	0	20	1	14	2	-
1 ea	Apple, medium	USDA	72	19	0	0	0	0	0	1	3	14	1	-
								SILVER						
1 c	Cottage Cheese, low-fat	Nancy's	160	6	28	2	1	0	10	608	0	6	-	-
1 serv	Yogurt, low-fat	Nancy's	150	16	11	3	3	0	20	170	0	16	-	-
1 c	Non-fat Cottage Cheese	Cabot	140	10	26	0	0	0	10	820	0	9	-	-
								BRONZE						
6 oz.	Yogurt, plain	Nancy's	130	11	8	6	4	0	25	125	0	11	-	-
1 c	Cottage Cheese	Cabot	200	8	26	9	6	-	30	800	0	8	-	-

ZERO-VALUE - does not apply

MEAL: BREAKFAST   GROUP: 9   CATEGORY: TOASTER/MICROWAVE

SELECTION TIPS: The amount of sodium is an issue with all frozen products. Look for **fiber** to be at least 3 grams. Limiting the amount of total **fat** and **saturated fat** are also a major consideration for these products.

Amt	Food	Brand	Kcal	CHO	PRO	FAT	Sat Fat	Trans Fat	Chol	Sodium	Fiber	Sugar	Fruit	Veggie
								GOLD						
2 ea	Waffles, frozen	Kashi	170	33	8	3	0	0	0	330	6	4	-	-
1 ea	Breakfast Burrito, black bean	Amy's Kitchen	210	38	9	6	0	0	0	540	5	4	-	-
2 ea	Waffles, low-fat	Eggo	142	28	4	2	0	-	0	430	3	4	-	-
								SILVER						
2 ea	Eggo, whole wheat	Eggo	180	28	5	6	1	1	0	420	3	3	-	-
2 ea	Waffles, frozen	Flax Plus	240	30	5	9	1	0	0	420	4	5	-	-
								BRONZE						
1 ea	Pastry, cherry	Pop Tarts	204	38	2	5	1	-	0	220	1	17	-	-
1 ea	Breakfast Hot Pocket	Hot Pockets	300	18	7	8	3	0	17	310	2	4	-	-
								ZERO-VALUE						
1 serv	Breakfast Burrito, bacon	Swanson's	250	27	10	11	4	-	90	540	1	3	-	-
1 ea	Sandwich, sausage	Jimmy Dean	192	12	4.7	14	4.3	-	16	440	0.7	-	-	-
1 ea	Hot Pockets, sausage	Hot Pockets	370	40	11	18	8	-	40	540	20	90	-	-

MEAL: BREAKFAST		GROUP: 10						CATEGORY: PASTRY/BAKERY							

SELECTION TIPS: These items have no place as an everyday breakfast choice. You are not going to find any Gold products for this category. You will have to look long and hard for a few foods ranked Silver. Most of these pastry and bakery items are going to be Bronze and Zero-Value. It is possible to find a fairly healthy muffin if you look hard enough.

Amt	Food	Brand	Kcal	CHO	PRO	FAT	Sat Fat	Trans Fat	Chol	Sodium	Fiber	Sugar	Fruit	Veggie
								GOLD - does not apply						
								SILVER						
1 ea	Scone, fat-free, cranberry	Health Valley	180	43	4	0	0	0	0	190	5	18	-	-
1 ea	Muffin, bran, low fat	Dunkin Donuts	260	59	4	1.5	0	-	0	440	4	33	-	-
								BRONZE						
1 ea	Scone, whole wheat	USDA	144	18	5	7	2	-	50	175	3	2	-	-
1 ea	Muffin, oat bran	USDA	270	48	7	7	1	0	0	393	5	8	-	-
1 ea	Donut, glazed, 3-inch	USDA	125	14	2	7	2	-	2	106	0	7	-	-
1 ea	Cupcake, choc	Tastykake	110	19	2	3	1	-	5	135	1	12	-	-
								ZERO-VALUE						
1 ea	Pastry, cheese swirl	Entenmanns	500	68	10	20	6	-	70	500	2	36	-	-
1 ea	Donut, glazed, 5-inch	USDA	492	54	8	28	7	-	7	417	1	29	-	-
1 ea	Ding Dong	Hostess	368	45	3	19	11	-	14	241	2	32	-	-
1 ea	Croissant, choc.	USDA	234	25	5	14	8	-	38	376	2	32	-	-

MEAL: LUNCH   GROUP: 11   CATEGORY: SANDWICH MEAT

SELECTION TIPS: Most selections are going to be a good source of **protein**. However, many items are high in **fat, saturated fat,** and **sodium**. Fresh turkey and chicken will have less sodium. Also check for the amount of fat in products containing mayonnaise.

Amt	Food	Brand	Kcal	CHO	PRO	FAT	Sat Fat	Trans Fat	Chol	Sodium	Fiber	Sugar	Fruit	Veggie
						GOLD								
4 oz.	Tuna, in water, can	USDA	145	0	27	3.4	1	-	48	427	0	0	-	-
2 tbsp	Peanut Butter	USDA	188	6.9	7.7	16	2.6	-	0	5.4	2.6	2.7	-	-
						SILVER								
4 oz.	Virginia Ham	Healthy Choice	120	2	18	3	1	-	50	840	0	2	-	-
4 oz.	Turkey Breast	Oscar Mayer	107	3.9	18	1.9	1	-	3.9	1330	0	0.2	-	-
4 oz.	Chicken Breast	Louis Rich	111	4.2	22	0.6	0.18	-	59	1294	0	0.8	-	-
4 oz.	Roast Beef	USDA	120	4	20	2	1	-	40	840	0	0	-	-
						BRONZE								
4 oz.	Tuna Salad	USDA	295	10	14	21	3.5	-	34	657	2.8	4.5	-	-
4 oz.	Cheese	Sara Lee	320	0	20	28	24	-	60	1120	0	0	-	-
1 serv	Spam, pork & ham	Hormel	176	1.7	7.5	15	5.6	-	40	776	0	-	-	-
2 serv	Bologna	Oscar Mayer	179	1.4	6.3	16.5	7.3	-	36	668	0	0.8	-	-

ZERO-VALUE - does not apply

| MEAL: LUNCH | | GROUP: 12 | | | | | | | CATEGORY: SANDWICH BREAD | | | |

SELECTION TIPS: The easiest way to pick healthy bread is to look at the **fiber** content (3-4 grams per serving is good). Also look for the words "whole wheat" or "whole grain" or "100% whole wheat flour" listed first on the ingredients list.

Amt	Food	Brand	Kcal	CHO	PRO	FAT	Sat Fat	Trans Fat	Chol	Sodium	Fiber	Sugar	Fruit	Veggie
						GOLD								
1 pc.	Whole Grain bread	Natural Ovens	60	14	2	1	0	0	0	80	5	1	-	-
1 pc.	Pita, Whole Wheat	USDA	170	35	6.3	1.7	0.3	-	0	340	4.7	0.5	-	-
1 pc.	Multigrain 100%	Sara Lee	80	14	4	1	0	0	0	135	4	3	-	-
						SILVER								
1 pc.	Pumpernickel	USDA	80	15.2	2.8	1	0.1	-	0	214	2.1	0.2	-	-
1 pc.	Rye	Pepperidge Farm	80	15	3	1	0	-	0	210	2	1	-	-
1 pc.	Seven Grain	Oroweat	100	20	3	1	0	0	0	180	2	4	-	-
						BRONZE								
1 pc.	White	Pepperidge Farm	65	11.5	2	1.2	0.5	-	0	130	0.5	1.5	-	-
1 pc.	Pita, white	USDA	77	15.6	2.5	0.3	0	-	0	150	0.6	0.4	-	-
						ZERO-VALUE - does not apply								

MEAL: LUNCH   GROUP: 13   CATEGORY: CONDIMENTS

SELECTION TIPS: Keep close watch on the serving sizes and the amount of **fat** for all mayonnaise and oily products. It is quite easy to ruin a perfectly healthy meal with the wrong choice of condiments.

Amt	Food	Brand	Kcal	CHO	PRO	FAT	Sat Fat	Trans Fat	Chol	Sodium	Fiber	Sugar	Fruit	Veggie
							GOLD							
1 tbsp	Mustard	Hebrew National	12	0	0	0	0	0	0	195	0	0	-	-
1 tbsp	Ketchup	USDA	14.5	3.8	0.3	0.1	0	-	0	167	0	3.4	-	-
1 tbsp	Miracle Whip, fat free	Kraft	13	2.5	0.03	0.4	0.1	-	1.4	126	0.3	1.6	-	-
1 tbsp	Mayonnaise, fat free	USDA	11	1.9	0.03	0.4	0.1	-	1.6	120	0.3	1.1	-	-
							SILVER							
1 tbsp	Mayonnaise, light	USDA	50	1.3	0.1	4.9	0.7	-	5.2	119	0	0.6	-	-
1 tbsp	Miracle Whip	Kraft	45	2	0	4	0.5	-	0	0.16	0	0.4	-	-
							BRONZE							
1 tbsp	Mayonnaise, real	Hellmann's	100	0	0	11	1.5	-	5	90	0	0	-	-
1 tbsp	Oil & Vinegar	USDA	70	0	0	7.8	1.4	-	0	0.16	0	0.6	-	-
1 tbsp	Mayonnaise, canola	USDA	100	0	0	11	0.5	0	5	90	0	0	-	-
							ZERO-VALUE							
1/4 tsp	Table salt	USDA	0	0	0	0	0	0	0	581	0	0	-	-

SELECTION TIPS: You just need to use some common sense to choose properly. Fruits and vegetables are going to be better than fries and chips. Small fries are better than large fries. Products with mayonnaise should be limited or avoided. It's that simple!

Amt	Food	Brand	Kcal	CHO	PRO	FAT	Sat Fat	Trans Fat	Chol	Sodium	Fiber	Sugar	Fruit	Veggie
						GOLD								
1 c	Fruit Salad, citrus	USDA	99	25	0.9	0.56	0.14	0	0	0.74	3.3	-	0.7	-
1 c	4 Bean Salad	USDA	100	19	4	0.5	0	-	0	300	3	8	-	0.2
1 c	Cucumber Salad	USDA	100	26	2	0	0	0	0	1160	-	20	0	1.5
						SILVER								
3	Pickle Spears, dill	USDA	12.6	2.7	0.63	0.15	0.04	0	0	918	1.2	1.4	-	0.8
1 c	Fruit Salad, heavy syrup	USDA	186	48.7	0.87	0.18	0.03	0	0	153	2.5	46	1	-
						BRONZE								
1 c	Cole Slaw	USDA	94	14.5	1.5	3.1	0.46	-	9.6	27.6	1.8	-	-	1.3
½ c	Potato Salad	USDA	166	23.4	1.5	7.6	1.1	-	3.7	454	1.5	8.3	-	0.6
½ c	Macaroni Salad	USDA	219	22.7	3	12.8	1.89	-	11.3	401	1.5	8.3	-	0.2
						ZERO-VALUE								
Small	French Fries	USDA	271	31.9	3.2	14.5	3.4	3.7	0	164	2.9	0.6	-	0.8
1 oz.	Potato Chips	USDA	130	19	2	5	0.5	-	-	19	80	0	0	1

	MEAL: LUNCH	GROUP: 15											CATEGORY: PIZZA	

SELECTION TIPS: Must check on serving sizes. The size of a slice of pizza varies greatly. Watch the amount of **saturated fat.** Also look for higher amounts of **fiber**. Fiber can range from 1 to 5 grams per slice.

Amt	Food	Brand	Kcal	CHO	PRO	FAT	Sat Fat	Trans Fat	Chol	Sodium	Fiber	Sugar	Fruit	Veggie
						GOLD								
1 pc.	Vegetable, French bread	Healthy Choice	280	44	17	4	1.5	-	10	480	5	8	-	1
1 pc	Mushroom, olive, 1/3 whole	Amy's Kitchen	250	33	10	9	3	-	10	560	2	3	-	0.1
1 pc.	Cheese, French bread	Lean Cuisine	310	48	16	6	3.5	-	15	520	4	5	-	0.1
						SILVER								
1 pc.	Cheese	Papa John's	304	38	13	11	4.5	-	22.2	676	2.2	6.2	-	0.1
1 pc.	Cheese	Little Caesar's	268	31	13	10.4	4.3	-	23.5	440	1.3	3.7	-	0.1
						BRONZE								
1 pc.	5 Cheese, tomato	California Pizza Kitchen	320	29	18	15	9	-	35	720	1	6	-	0.3
1 pc.	Cheese, ¾ of whole	Celeste	317	27.8	14.2	16.6	7	-	20	770	2.2	-	-	0.1
1 pc.	Cheese, deluxe for one	Celeste	582	51.2	22.7	31.8	10	-	20	1367	4.4	-	-	0.3
						ZERO-VALUE - does not apply								

| MEAL: LUNCH | | GROUP: 16 | | | | | | | | CATEGORY: MICROWAVE ITEMS | | | |

SELECTION TIPS: Be on the look-out for the amount of **fat** and **saturated fat**. Also be aware of the high **salt** content of many frozen foods. These products should not be eaten on a regular basis.

Amt	Food	Brand	Kcal	CHO	PRO	FAT	Sat Fat	Trans Fat	Chol	Sodium	Fiber	Sugar	Fruit	Veggie
								GOLD - does not apply						
								SILVER						
1 ea.	Pizza, pocket, pepperoni	Lean Pockets	290	45	13	7	2.5	-	30	600	2	4	-	-
1 ea.	Cheese Enchilada	Banquet	360	56	12	10	4	-	20	1500	8	7	-	-
1 ea.	Chicken Burrito	USDA	517	74	27	12	2.29	-	45	1399	5.7	-	-	-
1 serv	Sandwich, turkey, ham, cheese	Hot Pocket	310	43	14	10	4.5	-	40	730	2	13	-	-
								BRONZE						
1 serv	Pizza, 4 cheese	Hot Pocket	370	43	13	16	9	-	50	620	2	15	-	-
1 ea.	Fish Cake w/ potato	USDA	450	35	28	22.1	6.1	-	91	1965	5.2	-	-	0.9
								ZERO-VALUE						
1 ea.	Macaroni & Cheese	Stouffer's	680	64	26	36	16	-	60	1960	4	10	-	-

		MEAL: DINNER		GROUP: 17				CATEGORY: APPETIZERS							

SELECTION TIPS: Appetizers typically aren't very healthy. Best to have soup, salad, or vegetables (with a health dip) before meals. Try to avoid fried anything.

Amt	Food	Brand	Kcal	CHO	PRO	FAT	Sat Fat	Trans Fat	Chol	Sodium	Fiber	Sugar	Fruit	Veggie
						GOLD - does not apply								
						SILVER - does not apply								
						BRONZE								
1 serv	Stuffed Mushrooms	USDA	137	13	5.2	7.3	2.18	0	6.11	297	0.89	2.8	-	-
1 ea.	Vegetable Roll	USDA	158	19	4.2	6.9	0.92	-	2.8	262	0.95	0.35	-	-
1 ea.	Egg Roll, no meat	USDA	100	9.8	2.5	5.8	1.2	-	30	274	0.82	-	-	-
2 ea.	Deviled Eggs	USDA	125	0.78	7.2	10.1	2.47	-	243	100	0	0.74	-	-
4 ea.	Buffalo Wings	USDA	200	6.3	22	9.7	2.6	-	102	701	0.88	5.04	-	-
½ ea.	Cheese Quesadilla	USDA	270	25.5	11	13	7	-	30	588	1	0.5	-	-
1 serv	Fried Calamari	USDA	149	6.6	15.2	6.3	1.6	-	221	260	0	-	-	-
						ZERO-VALUE								
1 serv	Nachos, bean & cheese, large	USDA	501	49	17.4	27	11	-	18	1588	-	-	-	-
1 serv	Fried Mozzarella Sticks	USDA	290	25	12	16	6	-	20	670	1	1	-	-
1 serv	Fried Zucchini	USDA	340	37	5	19	4.5	-	0	860	2	2	-	0.31

MEAL: DINNER   GROUP: 18   CATEGORY: SOUP

SELECTION TIPS: Be careful with all "cream" soups that are high in total **fat** and **saturated fat**. Also beware of the high **sodium** levels. Also check for the number of servings per can. One small can of soup is usually 2 or 2.5 servings.

Amt	Food	Brand	Kcal	CHO	PRO	FAT	Sat Fat	Trans Fat	Chol	Sodium	Fiber	Sugar	Fruit	Veggie
						GOLD								
1 c	Chucky Tomato, fat-free	Health Valley	80	18	3	0	0	0	0	380	2	11	-	0.32
1 c	Black Bean	Campbell's	220	38	10	4	0	-	0	1800	10	8	-	0.29
						SILVER								
1 c	Chicken Noodle	Campbell's	100	16	9	2.5	1	-	20	860	2	3	-	-
1 c	Beef Barley	Progresso	142	20	11.3	1.9	0.75	-	19.2	469	3.1	-	-	0.23
						BRONZE								
1 c	Cream of Chicken, fat-free	Campbell's	140	20	6	4	2	-	20	1780	2	2	-	-
1 c	Chicken Gumbo	Campbell's	120	20	4	2	1	-	10	1740	2	4	-	-
1 c	Bean w/ Bacon	Campbell's	340	50	16	8	3	-	10	1720	16	8	-	-
						ZERO-VALUE								
10.7 oz.	Broccoli, cheese	USDA	265	23.4	6.4	16.2	4.9	-	12.2	2083	5.49	6.47	-	0.38
10.7 oz.	Cream of Chicken	USDA	284	22.5	8.36	17.9	5.04	-	23.7	2395	0.59	-	-	-
1 serv	Cream of Mushroom	USDA	314	22.5	5.6	21.87	5.9	-	5.9	2140	1.19	3.56	-	-

MEAL: DINNER

GROUP: 19

CATEGORY: MEAT

SELECTION TIPS: Great sources of **protein** but need to watch the amount of **fat** and **saturated fat**. Keep in mind that the serving sizes of the examples below are not equal.

Amt	Food	Brand	Kcal	CHO	PRO	FAT	Sat Fat	Trans Fat	Chol	Sodium	Fiber	Sugar	Fruit	Veggie
						GOLD								
1 ea.	Ground Beef Patty, 5% fat	USDA	140	0	21.5	5.37	2.4	0.14	62	53	0	0	-	-
6 oz.	Top Sirloin, lean	USDA	302	0	50	9.9	3.78	-	93	103	0	0	-	-
						SILVER								
1 ea.	Ground Beef Patty, 20% fat	USDA	208	0	19.8	13.7	5.2	0.95	70	57	0	0	-	-
6 oz.	Veal Chop, lion	USDA	297	0	44.7	11.8	4.39	-	180	163	0	0	-	-
6 oz.	Ham, baked	USDA	152	0	29	3.98	1.38	-	70	2050	0	0	-	-
						BRONZE								
6 oz.	Pork Chop, lion	USDA	421	0	46	24	9.13	-	139	100	0	0	-	-
6 oz.	T-Bone steak	USDA	439	0	41	29.3	10.9	-	103	113	0	0	-	-
1 ea.	Hot Dog, beef	USDA	180	3	6	16	7	-	35	620	0	0	-	-
						ZERO-VALUE								
6 oz.	Pork Sausage	USDA	585	7.2	32.5	46.45	16.2	-	142	1274	0	0	-	-
6 oz.	Ribs, roasted	USDA	629	0	41	50.3	18.6	-	200	171	0	0	-	-

MEAL: DINNER		GROUP: 20			CATEGORY: POULTRY									

SELECTION TIPS: Choose products without skin to limit fat intake. Fried anything should be avoided. Watch for the amount of total **fat** and **saturated fat**.

Amt	Food	Brand	Kcal	CHO	PRO	FAT	Sat Fat	Trans Fat	Chol	Sodium	Fiber	Sugar	Fruit	Veggie
						GOLD								
1 ea.	Chicken Breast, w/o skin, broiled	USDA	129	0	27.2	1.4	0.39	0.03	68	76	0	0	-	-
1 ea.	Duck Breast, w/o skin	USDA	133	0	26.2	2.3	0.5	-	135	99	0	0	-	-
1 ea.	Turkey Breast w/o skin	Boston Market	170	3	36	1	0	-	100	850	0	3	-	-
						SILVER								
1 ea.	Chicken Breast w/ skin	USDA	187	0	30	7	2	-	128	540	0	0	-	-
1 ea.	Chicken Drumstick	USDA	117	0	14	6.3	1.7	-	59	605	0	0	-	-
1 ea.	Turkey Patty	USDA	153	0	19.2	8.5	2.07	-	70	450	0	0	-	-
						BRONZE								
¾ ea.	Chicken, rotisserie w/ skin	Boston Market	280	2	40	12	3.5	-	135	510	0	2	-	-
1 serv	Chicken, breaded and fried	USDA	190	10.4	9.9	12	2.5	-	35.2	367	0.58	0.56	-	-
1 ea.	Chicken Patty	Country Skillet	190	12	9	11	2.5	-	20	490	1	3	-	-
4 ea.	Chicken Tenders	Country Skillet	179	10.7	10.7	10.3	2.6	2.01	32.2	447	1.4	0.07	-	-
					ZERO-VALUE - does not apply									

MEAL: DINNER GROUP: 21 CATEGORY: SEAFOOD

SELECTION TIPS: Salmon, halibut, and mackerel are good sources of Omega-3 fatty acids known to be healthy for the heart. Most seafood is healthy, but you must be careful of cooking methods and the use of excess butter, frying, or breading.

Amt	Food	Brand	Kcal	CHO	PRO	FAT	Sat Fat	Trans Fat	Chol	Sodium	Fiber	Sugar	Fruit	Veggie
						GOLD								
3 oz.	Salmon, chinook, broiled	USDA	196	0	21.8	11.3	2.7	-	72	51	0	0	-	-
3 oz.	Halibut, broiled	USDA	119	0	22.7	2.5	0.35	-	35	58	0	0	-	-
3 oz.	Mackerel, broiled	USDA	222	0	20	15	3.5	-	64	70	0	0	-	-
3 oz.	Tuna, cooked	USDA	131	0	26	1.5	0	0	50	40	0	0	-	-
						SILVER								
3 oz.	Fish Sticks, breaded	USDA	211	18	9.3	11.2	2.35	0.73	27	358	0	0	-	-
3 oz.	Shrimp, breaded	USDA	205	21.2	8.3	9.8	1.5	-	27	463	0	0	-	-
3 oz.	Lobster, stemmed	USDA	83	1.09	17.4	0.5	0.09	-	61	323	0	0	-	-
3 oz.	Scallops, steamed	USDA	95	0	19.7	1.19	0.12	-	45	225	0	0	-	-
3 oz.	Shrimp, steamed	USDA	101	0	21.2	105	0	0	172	242	0	0	-	-
						BRONZE								
3 oz.	Lobster, w/ butter	USDA	203	0	13.6	16	9.8	-	90	409	0	0	-	-
3 oz.	Scallops, fried	USDA	227	22.7	9.3	11.4	2.8	-	64	542	0	0	-	-

ZERO-VALUE - does not apply

MEAL: DINNER   GROUP: 22   CATEGORY: MEAT SUBSTITUES

SELECTION TIPS: Meat substitutes are good sources of **protein**. Protein sources from beans need to be combined (within the same day) with a complimentary protein, such as rice, to supply a complete protein.

Amt	Food	Brand	Kcal	CHO	PRO	FAT	Sat Fat	Trans Fat	Chol	Sodium	Fiber	Sugar	Fruit	Veggie
								GOLD						
4 oz.	Tofu, extra firm	USDA	100	2.8	10	5.7	0	0	0	0	1.4	0	-	-
3 ea.	Egg whites, cooked	USDA	50	1.03	10.5	0	0	0	0	164	0	0	-	-
2 tbsp	Peanut Butter	USDA	188	6.9	7.7	15.9	2.59	-	0	155	2.5	2.6	-	-
1 ea.	Veggie Burger	Morningstar	110	9.6	11.9	2.7	0.38	-	1.34	349	2.9	0.97	-	-
1 ea.	Soy Veggie Burger	Morningstar	132	12	13	3.5	0	-	0	330	7	4	-	-
1 ea.	Chicken Soy Burger	Yves Veggie Cuisine	110	6	15	2.8	0	-	0	280	2	0	-	-
1 c	Lentils, cooked	USDA	229	40	17.8	0.75	0.1	0	0	3.96	15.6	3.5	-	-
1 c	Garbanzo beans, cooked	USDA	268	44	14.5	4.25	0.44	0	0	11.5	12.4	7.8	-	-
								SILVER						
3 ea.	Whole eggs fried in oil	USDA	363	0.4	19.3	31.6	7	-	589	289	0	0.4	-	-
								BRONZE - does not apply						
								ZERO-VALUE - does not apply						

MEAL: DINNER   GROUP: 23   CATEGORY: VEGETABLES/LEGUMES (STARCHY)

SELECTION TIPS: All are excellent food choices. The only way to go wrong is to eat too much or to use too much butter or salt.

Amt	Food	Brand	Kcal	CHO	PRO	FAT	Sat Fat	Trans Fat	Chol	Sodium	Fiber	Sugar	Fruit	Veggie
						GOLD								
1 ea.	Baked Potato, small	USDA	128	29	3.4	0.18	0.05	0	0	13.7	3	1.6	-	1.13
½ c	Corn, white	USDA	67	13.4	2.2	0.75	0	-	0	0	2.2	-	-	0.63
½ c	Peas, frozen	USDA	62	11.4	4.12	0.22	0.04	0	0	258	4.4	3.7	-	0.5
½ c	Carrots	USDA	27	6.4	0.59	0.14	0.02	0	0	45	2.3	2.6	-	0.5
1 ea.	Baked Yam, medium	USDA	103	23.6	2.29	0.17	0.06	0	0	280	3.7	9.6	-	0.93
½ c	Squash, acorn, cubed	USDA	57	14.9	1.15	0.14	0.03	0	0	246	4.5	3.6	-	0.5
1 ea.	Sweet Potato, medium	USDA	102	23.6	2.29	0.17	0.03	0	0	41	3.7	7.39	-	0.93
½ c	Black Beans	USDA	113	20.4	7.6	0.46	0.12	0	0	203	7.48	-	-	-
½ c	Pinto Beans	USDA	122	22.4	7.7	0.56	0.09	0	0	203	7.6	0.29	-	-
½ c	Lentils	USDA	112	19.3	8.9	0.38	0.05	0	0	235	7.8	1.7	-	-
½ c	Hummus Spread	USDA	207	17.8	9.8	12	1.8	0	0	473	7.5	-	-	-

SILVER - does not apply

BRONZE - does not apply

ZERO-VALUE - does not apply

MEAL: DINNER   GROUP: 24   CATEGORY: VEGETABLES (NON-STARCHY)

SELECTION TIPS: All are excellent food choices. The only way to go wrong is to eat too much or use too much butter, salt, or salad dressing.

Amt	Food	Brand	Kcal	CHO	PRO	FAT	Sat Fat	Trans Fat	Chol	Sodium	Fiber	Sugar	Fruit	Veggie
						GOLD								
1 c	Broccoli	USDA	54	11.2	3.7	0.64	0.12	0	0	64	5.15	2.17	-	1
1 c	Cauliflower	USDA	34	6.7	2.9	0.4	0.06	0	0	32.4	4.8	1.89	-	1.4
1 c	Green Beans	USDA	25	4	1	0	0	0	0	10	2	2	-	0.49
1 c	Spinach	USDA	20	3	2	0	0	0	0	115	2	1	-	0.45
1 c	Cabbage	USDA	34	8.3	1.9	0.09	0	0	0	382	2.8	4.2	-	1
1 c	Zucchini	USDA	28	7.07	1.15	0.09	0.02	-	0	5.4	2.5	3.04	-	0.85
1 c	Asparagus	USDA	39	7.4	4.3	0.4	0.09	0	0	432	3.6	2.3	-	0.74
1 c	Eggplant, cooked	USDA	34	8.64	0.82	0.23	0.04	0	0	0.99	2.47	3.17	-	1
½ ea.	Avocado (fruit)	USDA	160	8.57	2.01	14.7	2.14	0	0	7	6.7	0.66	1	-
1 c	Mushrooms	USDA	43.6	8.2	3.39	0.73	0.08	0	0	3.12	3.4	3	-	1
2 c	Lettuce, Romaine	USDA	19	3.7	1.38	0.34	0.04	0	0	8.9	2.3	1.3	-	1
2 c	Lettuce. Iceberg	USDA	15.4	3.27	0.99	0.15	0.02	0	0	11	1.27	2	-	0.98
½ c	Tomato, plum	USDA	16.2	3.53	0.79	0.18	0.03	0	0	4.5	1.08	2.37	-	0.5
1 serv	Celery	USDA	6.4	1.19	0.28	0.07	0.02	0	0	32	0.58	0.61	-	0.33
½ c	Cucumber	USDA	7.8	1.89	0.34	0.06	0.02	0	0	1.04	0.26	0.87	-	0.43
1 c	Red Peppers, cooked	USDA	38	9.1	1.25	0.27	0.04	0	0	2.7	1.6	4.6	-	1
						SILVER - does not apply								
						BRONZE - does not apply								
						ZERO-VALUE - does not apply								

MEAL: DINNER   GROUP: 25   CATEGORY: GRAINS/RICE

SELECTION TIPS: A good source of **carbohydrates**. Having the proper amount is the key as well as not adding too much butter or salt.

Amt	Food	Brand	Kcal	CHO	PRO	FAT	Sat Fat	Trans Fat	Chol	Sodium	Fiber	Sugar	Fruit	Veggie
						GOLD								
½ c	Brown Rice, Long Grain	USDA	108	22	2.5	0.8	0.18	0	0	4.8	1.75	0.34	-	-
½ c	Wild Rice	USDA	82	17.5	3.27	0.28	0.04	0	0	2.4	1.48	0.6	-	-
½ c	Couscous	USDA	88	18.2	2.9	0.13	0.02	0	0	3.9	1.1	0.08	-	-
						SILVER								
½ c	White Rice	USDA	120	26.5	2.21	0.2	0.05	0	0	2.2	0.28	0.46	-	-
1 serv	White Rice, Long Grain	USDA	102	22.2	2.13	0.22	0.06	0	0	301	0.32	0.04	-	-
1 serv	Stuffing, bread	USDA	100	19	3	1	0	-	0	405	1	0	-	-
1 serv	Stuffing, cornbread	Uncle Ben's	100	21	3	1	0	0	0	490	1	3	-	-
1 serv	Stuffing, cornbread	Stove Top	106	20.4	3.5	1.15	0.22	-	1.12	428	0.7	2.8	-	-
						BRONZE								
1 serv	Stuffing, chicken	Stove top	120	19	3	3	0	0	0	460	1	2	-	-
1 serv	Rice Pilaf	USDA	140	24	2	4	0.5	-	0	520	1	2	-	-

ZERO-VALUE - does not apply

| MEAL: DINNER | | GROUP: 26 | | | | | | | | | CATEGORY: SALAD DRESSING | | | | |

SELECTION TIPS: Check the serving size and limit the amount of **calories** and **saturated fat**. A fine balance is needed: you don't want to use too much dressing and negate the health benefits of the salad, but you also want the salad to taste good. It's worth finding a low calorie/low fat dressing that you like.

Amt	Food	Brand	Kcal	CHO	PRO	FAT	Sat Fat	Trans Fat	Chol	Sodium	Fiber	Sugar	Fruit	Veggie
						GOLD								
2 tbsp	French, fat-free	USDA	42	10.3	0.06	0.09	0.01	-	0	255	0.7	5.26	-	-
2 tbsp	Catalina, fat-free	Kraft	35	8	0	0	0	0	0	320	1	7	-	-
						SILVER								
2 tbsp	Balsamic Vinaigrette	Organic Spectrum	80	3	0	8	0	0	0	230	0	2	-	-
2 tbsp	Ranch, light	USDA	80	3	0	7	0.5	0	10	300	0	1	-	-
2 tbsp	Italian, reduced fat	Kraft	40	3	0	3	0.5	-	0	270	0	2	-	-
						BRONZE								
2 tbsp	Thousand Island	USDA	115	4.57	0.34	10.9	1.6	-	8.1	269	0.25	4.3	-	-
						ZERO-VALUE								
2 tbsp	Caesar	USDA	155	0.9	0.35	17	2.58	-	0.59	317	0.03	0.39	-	-
2 tbsp	Blue Cheese	Wishbone	170	2	1	17	3	-	10	280	0	-	-	-
2 tbsp	Oil & Vinegar	USDA	140	0.8	0	15.6	2.8	-	0	0.31	0	0.78	-	-

MEAL: DINNER GROUP: 27 CATEGORY: PASTA

SELECTION TIPS: It is very easy to overeat pasta. The most important column to watch is therefore **calories**. The amounts below are all based on one cup of cooked pasta. Also look for pastas with a high **fiber** content such as whole wheat pasta.

Amt	Food	Brand	Kcal	CHO	PRO	FAT	Sat Fat	Trans Fat	Chol	Sodium	Fiber	Sugar	Fruit	Veggie
						GOLD								
1 c	Spaghetti, whole wheat	USDA	173	37	7.46	0.76	0.14	-	0	4.2	6.3	1.12	-	-
1 c	Pasta, corn	USDA	176	39	3.68	1.02	0.14	-	0	3.68	6.7	-	-	-
1 c	Egg, spinach	USDA	211	38	8.06	2.51	0.58	-	52.8	19.2	3.68	0.64	-	-
						SILVER								
1 c	Spaghetti, enriched	USDA	219	42.8	8.12	1.3	0.25	0	0	183.4	2.5	0.78	-	-
1 c	Pasta, buckwheat	USDA	162	33	4.62	0.98	-	-	-	-	0.28	-	-	-
1 c	Pasta, egg	USDA	220	40.2	7.26	3.31	0.67	0.03	46.4	8	1.92	0.64	-	-
1 c	Shells, enriched	USDA	181	35.4	6.67	1.07	0.2	0	0	1.15	2.07	6.67	-	-
						BRONZE								
1 c	Pasta, rice	USDA	191	43.8	1.6	0.35	0.04	0	0	33.4	1.7	-	-	-
1 c	Ramen, noodles	USDA	153	20.2	3.3	6.5	1.65	-	0.21	801	1.16	-	-	-

ZERO-VALUE - does not apply

| MEAL: DINNER | | | | | | | GROUP: 28 | | | | | CATEGORY: PASTA SAUCES | |

SELECTION TIPS: Watch once again for the serving size. For many products the serving size is 4 oz., but many will often use one cup (8 oz.). Total **fat** and **saturated fat** are important nutrients to watch. Gold Ranking has 0g saturated fat, Silver 1g, Bronze >2g.

Amt	Food	Brand	Kcal	CHO	PRO	FAT	Sat Fat	Trans Fat	Chol	Sodium	Fiber	Sugar	Fruit	Veggie
						GOLD								
1 c	Chunky, Tomato	Muir Glen	100	24	4	1	0	-	0	640	0	10	-	0.99
1 c	Balsamic, roasted	Muir Glen	100	24	4	1	0	-	0	640	0	10	-	1.11
1 c	Italian Style, w/ vegetables	Healthy Choice	80	18	4	0	0	0	0	780	4	14	-	1
						SILVER								
1 serv	Italian, sausage	Prego	90	12	3	3.5	1	-	5	760	208	9.1	-	0.32
1 c	Tomato, olive oil	Ragu	180	18	4	9	1	-	0	1420	4	14	-	1
						BRONZE								
1 c	5-Cheese	Bertolli	180	22	8	6	2	-	10	1320	-	-	-	1
1 c	Fresh Mushroom	Prego	240	42	4	7	3	-	0	1120	6	28	-	0.9
1 c	Mini Meatball	Prego	300	40	8	12	4	-	20	1300	6	24	-	0.7
1 c	Beef & Mushroom	Prego	260	28	12	12	5	-	20	1320	4	20	-	0.75
						ZERO-VALUE								
1 c	Alfredo, classic	Ragu	440	12	4	40	14	-	100	1360	0	4	-	-

MEAL: DINNER									GROUP: 29			CATEGORY: MICROWAVE MEALS			

SELECTION TIPS: Look to keep **saturated fat** 3 grams or less. **Sodium** content is high for these products. Sodium levels fewer than 800mg are considered acceptable.

Amt	Food	Brand	Kcal	CHO	PRO	FAT	Sat Fat	Trans Fat	Chol	Sodium	Fiber	Sugar	Fruit	Veggie
						GOLD								
1 ea.	Chicken, country herb	Healthy Choice	320	44	18	8	3	-	45	540	3	23	-	-
1 ea.	Roasted Chicken, rice & mushroom	Lean Cuisine	330	49	23	5	1	-	40	740	4	5	-	0.6
1 ea.	Roasted Turkey w/ stuffing	Lean cuisine	320	43	23	6	1	-	30	840	6	11	-	0.5
1 ea.	Beef, w/ potatoes & peppers	Stouffer's	300	44	17	6	1.5	-	25	830	7	7	-	1.3
						SILVER								
1 ea.	Cheese Enchilada	Banquet	360	56	12	10	4	-	20	1500	8	7	-	-
1 ea.	Meatballs & Pasta	Lean Cuisine	440	64	25	9	3.5	-	35	820	7	12	-	0.6
1 ea.	Chicken Burrito	USDA	517	74	27	12	2.29	-	45	1399	5.7	-	-	-
						BRONZE								
1 ea.	Fish Cake w/ potato	USDA	450	35	28	22.1	6.1	-	91	1965	5.2	-	-	0.9
1 ea.	Chimichanga	USDA	500	56	13	24	8	-	20	1180	9	13	-	-
1 ea.	Macaroni & Cheese	Banquet	420	57	15	14	8	-	20	1330	5	7	-	-
1 ea.	Beef Tips w/ mushroom sauce	Marie Callender's	430	39	25	19	7	-	50	1620	6	11	-	-

ZERO-VALUE - does not apply

MEAL: DESSERTS   GROUP: 30   CATEGORY: FROZEN

SELECTION TIPS: Select low fat products. Fruit popsicles are going to be your best bet along with low fat frozen yogurt or sorbet.

Amt	Food	Brand	Kcal	CHO	PRO	FAT	Sat Fat	Trans Fat	Chol	Sodium	Fiber	Sugar	Fruit	Veggie
						GOLD								
1 ea.	Frozen Pop, fantastic fruity	GH Popsicles	50	13	0	0	0	0	0	5	0	10	-	-
1 ea.	Frozen Fudge Bar, fat free	Sweet Nothings	100	23	1	0	0	0	0	5	0	12	-	-
1 serv	Sorbet, coffee	USDA	80	22	0	0	0	0	0	85	0	22	-	-
						SILVER								
1 ea.	Ice Cream Cone, low fat	USDA	110	20	3	1.5	0.5	0	5	95	4	12	-	-
1 serv	Ice Cream, cherry vanilla, low fat	Healthy Choice	120	22	2	2	1	-	5	50	1	17	-	-
						BRONZE								
1 ea.	Creamsicle, orange	USDA	100	18	1	2.5	1.5	-	5	30	0	14	-	-
1 ea.	Fudge Bar	Julie's Organic	100	14	2	4.5	2.5	0	15	40	1	12	-	-
1 ea.	Frozen Yogurt Bar, chocolate coated	USDA	109	11.8	1.32	6.7	5.34	-	0.64	28	0.1	10.1	-	-
						ZERO-VALUE								
1 ea.	Ice Cream Bar	Haagen Dazs	300	24	4	21	13	-	70	40	1	21	-	-
1 ea.	York Peppermint Patty bar	Klondike	280	24	3	19	13	-	20	55	1	20	-	-
1 ea.	Bar, coconut	Fruit-a-Freeze	200	25	2	11	8	0	20	55	1	12	-	-
1 ea.	Ice Cream Cone	Dairy Queen, Inc	340	53	8	11	7	-	30	160	0	34	-	-
1 serv	Ice Cream, choc.	Haagen Dazs	270	22	5	18	11	-	115	60	1	21	-	-

MEAL: DESSERTS GROUP: 31 CATEGORY: BAKERY

SELECTION TIPS: These items should be eaten occasionally or not at all. We eat these products because they taste good. But let's not kid ourselves; there are no nutrients in these products that we couldn't get from healthier sources. They certainly don't make it any easier to stay within our daily recommendations.

GOLD - does not apply

SILVER - does not apply

BRONZE - does not apply

ZERO-VALUE

Amt	Food	Brand	Kcal	CHO	PRO	FAT	Sat Fat	Trans Fat	Chol	Sodium	Fiber	Sugar	Fruit	Veggie
1 ea.	Ding-Dongs	Hostess	368	45.3	3.12	19.4	11	-	13.6	240	1.8	32.4	-	-
1 ea.	Doughnut, Boston Cream	Dunkin' Donuts	270	38	4	11	3	-	0	260	1	17	-	-
1 ea.	Cup Cake, chocolate	Tastykake	103	18.3	1.3	3.3	1	0.67	3.3	130	1	13	-	-
1 pc.	Coffee Cake, pecan Danish ring	Entenmann's	250	25	3	15	3	-	30	160	1	12	-	-
1 ea.	Éclair, custard filled	USDA	262	24	6.4	15.7	4.1	-	127	337	0.6	6.6	-	-
1 ea.	Cheesecake	Mrs. Smith's	510	40	9	36	-	-	155	330	-	28	-	-
1 ea.	Brownie, 2" square	USDA	111	12	1.49	6.9	1.7	-	17.5	82	0.53	-	-	-
1 ea.	Biscotti, almond	Perugina	127	18	1.06	5.3	2.1	-	26.5	48	1.1	9.5	-	-
1 pc.	Angel Food Cake	USDA	73	16.4	1.67	0.23	0.03	-	0	212	0.43	-	-	-
1 ea.	Sugar Cookie	USDA	72	10.1	0.76	3.2	0.82	-	7.6	53	0.12	5.6	-	-
1 pc.	Apple Pie	USDA	248	33.6	2.4	12	3.08	4.72	-	153	1.5	13.3	0.33	-

| MEAL: SNACK | GROUP: 32 | | | | | | | | | | | CATEGORY: ENERGY BARS |

SELECTION TIPS: Avoid bars that are low-**carb** (<10 grams/100kcal). Look for bars that can satisfy hunger and keep you feeling full, with >8 grams of **protein** and <3 grams of **saturated fat**. They are a major step up from candy bars. Good for a quick breakfast on the go, a convenient snack, or an occasional meal replacement. Cereal bars tend to be less filling being low in protein, but nevertheless a good snack.

Amt	Food	Brand	Kcal	CHO	PRO	FAT	Sat Fat	Trans Fat	Chol	Sodium	Fiber	Sugar	Fruit	Veggie
							GOLD - does not apply							
							SILVER							
1 ea.	Chocolate Brownie	Clif	236	40	10.4	4.2	1	-	0.11	149	5.6	20.2	-	-
1 ea.	Oatmeal Raisin Cookie	Kashi Go-Lean	280	49	13	5	3	0	0	110	0.78	-	-	-
1 ea.	Cereal, apple cobbler	Health Valley	130	27	2	2	0	-	0	50	1	13	-	-
1 ea.	Apple Cinnamon	Power Bar	230	45	10	2.5	0.5	0	0	90	3	20	-	-
1 ea.	Almond Brownie	Balance	200	21	15	7	2	0	0	140	2	17	-	-
1 ea.	Almond Raisin	Zone Perfect	210	23	15	7	3.5	0	5	250	<1	17	-	-
1 ea.	Chocolate	Myoplex Deluxe	340	45	10	2.5	0.5	0	0	140	2	17	-	-
1 ea.	Cereal, cherry	Nutri grain	136	27	1.6	2.7	0.55	-	0	110	0.78	-	-	-
							BRONZE							
1 ea.	Chocolate Coconut	Metabolift	120	7	12	4	2	-	-	80	5	2	-	-
1 ea.	Cereal, fruit & oatmeal	Quaker Oats	136	27	1.6	2.9	0.35	1.36	0.07	81	1	14	-	-
1 ea.	Caramel Crispy Peanut	Slim Fast	220	33	8	6	4	0	5	250	2	15	-	-
							ZERO-VALUE - does not apply							

MEAL: SNACK   GROUP: 33   CATEGORY: FRUITS/NUTS

SELECTION TIPS: You can't go wrong with this category as long as you don't overeat. Try to choose raw nuts and not nuts that roasted or salted. As always, be careful of **calorie** amounts. Dried fruit and nuts are very calorie dense.

Amt	Food	Brand	Kcal	CHO	PRO	FAT	Sat Fat	Trans Fat	Chol	Sodium	Fiber	Sugar	Fruit	Veggie
						GOLD								
1 ea.	Apple, medium	USDA	71	19	0.36	0.23	0.04	0	0	1.38	3.3	14.3	0.51	-
1 ea.	Banana, medium	USDA	105	27	1.29	0.39	0.13	0	0	1.18	3.07	14.4	0.48	-
½ ea.	Cantaloupe	USDA	138	33	3.4	0.77	0.21	0	0	65	3.6	29.6	2.3	-
½ c	Apricots, dried	Sunsweet	100	24	1	0	0	0	0	0	40	18	1.44	-
						SILVER								
1 oz.	Almonds (22 count)	USDA	164	5.6	6.22	14.3	1.1	0	0	7.9	2.9	1.4	-	-
1 oz.	Cashews (raw)	USDA	156	8.5	5.1	12.4	2.2	0	0	3.4	0.9	1.6	-	-
1 ea.	Raisins, small box	USDA	128	34	1.3	0.2	0.02	0	0	4.7	1.59	25.4	1.12	-
1 ea.	Bar, Trail Mix, fruit & nut	Nature Valley	140	25	3	4	0.5	0	0	95	2	13	-	-
½ c	Snack Mix, sweet & salty	Chex Mix	140	22	2	4.5	1.5	0	0	230	1.25	7	-	-
½ c	Mixed Tropical Fruit	Sunsweet	280	64	0	2	2	0	0	100	4	58	1.84	-
						BRONZE								
½ c	Trail Mix, tropical	USDA	284	45.9	4.4	11.9	5.9	-	0	7	4.4	-	1.11	-
½ c	Trail Mix, regular	USDA	346	33.6	10.3	22	4.2	-	0	7.5	3.85	-	1.48	-
½ c	Trail Mix, w/chocolate chips	USDA	350	32.5	10.3	23.1	4.4	-	2.9	87	4.02	-	-	-

ZERO-VALUE - does not apply

MEAL: SNACKS   GROUP: 34   CATEGORY: CHIPS/POPCORN

SELECTION TIPS: Very important to check the serving size. Most people typically eat much more than one serving. It is not uncommon for someone to eat the entire bag which can be more than 5 servings. So please double check the amounts that you are actually eating.

Amt	Food	Brand	Kcal	CHO	PRO	FAT	Sat Fat	Trans Fat	Chol	Sodium	Fiber	Sugar	Fruit	Veggie
						GOLD								
2 c	Popcorn, air popped	USDA	62	12.4	2	0.73	0.09	-	0	1.28	2.3	0.14	-	-
1 oz.	Tortilla Chips, blue corn	USDA	111	22	3	2	0	-	0	141	2	0	-	-
						SILVER								
1 ea.	Popcorn Cake	USDA	38.4	8	0.97	0.31	0.05	-						
1 ea.	Popcorn Cake, caramel apple	USDA	56	11.8	0.8	0.71	0.35	-	0.28	51	0.21	3.95	-	-
						BRONZE								
2 c	Buttered Popcorn	USDA	80	8.8	1.2	4.8	0.6	0	0	120	1.6	0.4	-	-
1 oz.	Tortilla, white corn	Tostitos	149	18	1	8	1	-	0	85	1	1	-	-
1 c	Cracker Jack's	Frito Lay	240	46	4	4	0	0	0	140	2	30	-	-
						ZERO-VALUE								
1 oz.	BBQ Potato Chips	Ruffles	159	15	2	10	2.5	-	0	319	1	1	-	1.01
1 ea.	Popcorn, cheese	USDA	115	11.3	2	7.3	1.4	-	2.4	195	2.1	-	-	-
1 oz.	Potato Crisps	Pringles	157	20.4	1.57	9.4	2.36	0	0	173	1.57	0	-	1.02
1 oz.	Potato Chips	USDA	155	14.1	1.8	10.6	3.11	-	0	148	1.25	0.1	-	1.01

MEAL: SNACKS   GROUP: 35   CATEGORY: DIPS

SELECTION TIPS: As always, glance at the **fat** and **saturated** fat content. Be aware of the **amounts** used.

Amt	Food	Brand	Kcal	CHO	PRO	FAT	Sat Fat	Trans Fat	Chol	Sodium	Fiber	Sugar	Fruit	Veggie
						GOLD								
2 tbsp	Salsa	USDA	10	2	0	0	0	0	0	160	0	1	-	0.1
2 tbsp	Bean Dip	Frito Lay	40	6	2	1	0.5	-	5	140	0	0	-	-
2 tbsp	Black Bean	Garden of Eatin	30	5	2	0	0	0	0	100	1	1	-	-
						SILVER								
2 tbsp	Guacamole	Kraft	50	3	1	4.5	2.5	0	0	240	0	1	-	-
						BRONZE								
2 tbsp	Cheese, light	Kraft	80	6	6	3.5	2	0	20	500	0	4	-	-
						ZERO-VALUE								
2 tbsp	Nacho Cheese	Kaukauna	90	4	3	7	2	-	10	330	0	3	-	-
2 tbsp	Cheese, original	USDA	90	4	3	7	4.5	-	30	490	0	3	-	-
2 tbsp	Sour Cream	USDA	60	20	1	5	3.5	0	20	10	1	1	-	-
2 tbsp	French Onion	USDA	50	1	1	5	3	-	15	190	0	1	-	-
2 tbsp	Ranch	USDA	50	1	1	5	3	-	15	160	0	1	-	-
2 tbsp	Vegetable Dip	Cabol	50	2	1	5	3	-	15	125	0	1	-	-
2 tbsp	Clam	USDA	50	1	1	5	3	-	15	120	0	0	-	-

MEAL: SNACKS		GROUP: 36									CATEGORY: CANDY			

SELECTION TIPS: All of these items merit a Zero-Value ranking.

Amt	Food	Brand	Kcal	CHO	PRO	FAT	Sat Fat	Trans Fat	Chol	Sodium	Fiber	Sugar	Fruit	Veggie
						GOLD - does not apply								
						SILVER - does not apply								
						BRONZE - does not apply								
						ZERO-VALUE								
2 oz.	Snicker's	Snicker's	475	60.5	7.5	23.8	9.1	0.44	13	246	2.3	50.5	-	-
2 oz.	5th Avenue	USDA	482	62.7	8.7	24	6.6	-	6	225	3.1	47.1	-	-
2.1 oz.	Baby Ruth	Baby Ruth	459	64.8	5.4	21.6	12.1	0.05	0	230	2	54	-	-
2.1 oz.	Butterfinger	Butterfinger	459	72.9	5.4	18.9	9.5	0.04	0	230	2	45.9	-	-
1.4 oz.	Chunky	Chunky	475	60	7.5	27.5	12.5	0.16	10	38	2.5	52.5	-	-
2 oz.	Heath	Heath	320	34.9	1.45	17.4	7.27	-	14.5	196	1.4	33.4	-	-
1.7 oz.	Almond Joy	Almond Joy	479	59.5	4.13	26.9	17.6	-	4	142	5	48.3	-	-
1.9 oz.	Reese's	Reese's	517	52.8	11.3	32.1	8.9	-	3	141	3.9	40.2	-	-
1.5 oz.	Crunch	Nestlé's	500	67	5	26	16	0.14	13	150	1.9	55	-	-
2.8 oz.	Kit Kat	USDA	518	64.6	6.5	25.9	17.9	0.1	11	54	1	46.8	-	-
2.1 oz.	Milky Way	Milky Way	452	70.4	4	17.2	12	0.21	9	167	1	59.6	-	-

MEAL: BEVERAGES GROUP: 37 CATEGORY: COLD

SELECTION TIPS: This category is easy. Drink plenty of water (roughly 64 oz. per day), 100% fruit juice, or vegetable juice (8 oz. per meal or snack). All soda, both diet and regular, should be limited or omitted from your diet. Also, you are asking for trouble if you consume too many of those high caffeinated (e.g, Red Bull) drinks. Choose non-fat or 1% milk instead of whole milk to reduce the **fat** and **saturated fat** content.

Amt	Food	Brand	Kcal	CHO	PRO	FAT	Sat Fat	Trans Fat	Chol	Sodium	Fiber	Sugar	Fruit	Veggie
	GOLD													
8 oz.	Skim (non-fat) milk	USDA	83.3	12.1	8.3	0.2	0.12	0	4.9	103	0	12.1	-	-
8 oz.	1% milk	USDA	102	12.2	8.2	2.4	1.5	-	12.2	107	0	12.2	-	-
8 oz.	Fresh orange juice	USDA	112	25.7	1.7	0.5	0.06	0	0	2.48	0.5	20.8	1	-
8 oz.	Soy Milk, low fat	Edensoy	100	15	5	2	0	0	0	90	0	10	-	-
8 oz.	Vegetable Juice, low-sodium	USDA	53	11.1	1.5	0.24	0.03	-	0	169	1.9	9.2	-	-
	SILVER													
8 oz.	2% Milk	USDA	122	11.4	8.1	4.8	3.1	0.15	19.5	100	1	11.4	-	-
8 oz.	Soy Milk, original	Edensoy	140	14	11	5	0.5	0	0	105	0.75	7	-	-
8 oz.	Vegetable Juice	V-8	50	11	2	0	0	0	0	460	2	8	-	-
	BRONZE													
8 oz.	Whole Milk	USDA	146	11	7.8	7.9	4.5	0.24	24.4	97.6	0	11	-	-
8 oz.	Chocolate Milk, 2%	USDA	190	30.3	7.47	4.75	2.9	0.15	20	165	1.7	23.9	-	-
	ZERO-VALUE													
8 oz.	Fruit Drink, 10% juice	Hi-C	98	26	0	0	0	0	0	133	0	26	-	-
8 oz.	Cola	Coca-Cola	103	26.7	0	0	0	0	0	5.3	0	26.7	-	-
8 oz.	Cola, diet	Coca-Cola	1	0.08	0	0	0	0	0	4	0	0.08	-	-
8 oz.	Sports Drink (not during activity)	Gatorade	62	15.1	0.24	0	0	0	0	94	0	12.8	-	-

MEAL: BEVERAGES   GROUP: 38   CATEGORY: ALCOHOL

SELECTION TIPS: All alcohol is Zero-Value, but that doesn't mean we are not going to drink it. We drink it because it tastes good and makes us feel good, not because we need the nutrients. Alcohol is not listed on the label as a standard **carbohydrate** or a **sugar**. Nevertheless, it still contains **calories** (about 7 kcal/gram). Red wine may have health benefits (due to resveratrol), but it still gets a Zero-Value ranking in my book.

Amt	Food	Brand	Kcal	CHO	PRO	FAT	Sat Fat	Trans Fat	Chol	Sodium	Fiber	Sugar	Fruit	Veggie
						GOLD - does not apply								
						SILVER - does not apply								
						BRONZE - does not apply								
						ZERO-VALUE								
5 oz.	Red Wine	USDA	123	3.69	0.1	0	0	0	0	5.8	0	0.91	-	-
5 oz.	White Wine	Pinot Grigio	123	3.02	0.1	0	0	0	-	-	-	-	-	-
12 oz.	Beer	Miller	143	13.1	1	0	0	0	0	7	-	-	-	-
12 oz.	Beer. Lite	Budweiser	96	3.6	0.8	0	0	0	0	9	-	-	-	-
12 oz.	Pina Colada	USDA	655	85	1.6	7.08	6.16	-	0	22.6	1.13	84.1	-	-
2 oz.	Bourbon, 80 proof	USDA	164	0	0	0	0	0	0	0.56	0	0	-	-
2 oz.	Vodka	USDA	128	0	0	0	0	0	0	0.56	0	0	-	-
1 ea.	Screwdriver	USDA	181	18.5	1.2	0.1	0.01	-	0	2.13	0.34	18.1	-	-
1 ea.	Daiquiri, frozen	USDA	429	15.7	0.23	0.23	0.02	-	0	11.5	0	15.7	-	-
1 ea.	Margarita, frozen	USDA	169	10.7	0.05	0.09	0.01	-	0	4.05	0.06	10	-	-

MEAL: FAST FOODS (BURGER)   GROUP: 39   CATEGORY: BREAKFAST

SELECTION TIPS: Once again, this is a category that you need to watch the amount of calories, fat, and saturated fat.

Amt	Food	Brand	Kcal	CHO	PRO	FAT	Sat Fat	Trans Fat	Chol	Sodium	Fiber	Sugar	Fruit	Veggie
							GOLD - does not apply							
							SILVER							
1 ea.	Eggs, scrambled	McDonald's	195	1.8	15.2	14.8	4.1	0.39	431	193	-	0.26	-	-
1 ea.	English Muffin w/ spread	McDonald's	140	25	4	2	0	-	0	210	1	1	-	-
1 ea.	Pancakes w/ margarine & syrup	McDonald's	600	104	9	17	3	-	20	770	0	40	-	-
1 ea.	Sandwich, egg w/ biscuit	Burger King	390	37	11	22	5	-	150	1020	1	4	-	-
							BRONZE							
1 ea.	Hash Browns	McDonald's	140	15	1	8	1.5	2	0	290	2	-	-	-
1 ea.	Burrito, sausage	McDonald's	296	24	13	17.1	6	1.2	172	762	1.2	1.4	-	-
1 ea.	Croissant w/bacon, egg, cheese	Burger King	340	26	15	20	7	2	155	890	1	-	-	-
1 ea.	Danish, apple	McDonald's	340	47	5	15	3	-	20	340	2	21	-	-
							ZERO-VALUE							
1 ea.	Deluxe Breakfast	McDonald's	1220	133	33	61	17	11	565	1980	5	-	-	-
1 ea.	Sweet Roll w/ icing	Burger King	440	51	6	23	6	-	25	710	1	20	-	-
1 ea.	Biscuit	Burger King	300	35	6	15	3.5	-	0	830	1	3	-	-
1 ea.	Sandwich, bacon, egg, cheese	Burger King	692	50	27	61	18	-	252	2129	1.3	5.3	-	-

MEAL: FAST FOODS (BURGER)   GROUP: 40   CATEGORY: MAIN ITEMS

SELECTION TIPS: Common sense can go a long way when it comes to fast foods. First of all, do not make fast food a regular part of your diet. You may have good intentions, but sooner or later you will order something loaded with **calories** and **fat**. You don't need me to tell you that the smaller size burgers are going to better for you than the huge ones.

Amt	Food	Brand	Kcal	CHO	PRO	FAT	Sat Fat	Trans Fat	Chol	Sodium	Fiber	Sugar	Fruit	Veggie
	GOLD													
1 ea.	Salad, charbroiled chicken w/o dressing	Carl's Jr.	250	14	29	9	3.5	-	75	590	4	8	-	1.31
1 ea.	Chicken Sandwich w/o mayonnaise	McDonald's	350	45	26	7	1.5	-	50	890	2	7	-	0.09
1 ea.	Salad, Caesar w/chicken	McDonald's	213	11	29	6.14	3.03	0.16	72	858	3.3	4.8	-	1.96
1 ea.	Chicken, grilled	Wendy's	300	36	24	7	1.5	0	55	740	2	8	-	0.31
	SILVER													
1 ea.	Hamburger	Burger King	290	30	15	12	4.5	0	40	560	1	-	-	-
1 ea.	Cheeseburger	McDonald's	313	33	15.4	14	5.28	0.77	41.6	744	1.31	7.4	-	-
1 ea.	Cheeseburger Jr.	Wendy's	330	32.2	16.8	14.8	6.68	0.6	46.4	851	1.81	6.02	-	0.12
	BRONZE													
1 ea.	Filet o Fish	McDonald's	400	40.3	14.8	20.4	3.66	1.01	39.5	633	1.27	8.4	-	-
1 ea.	Chicken Sandwich	Carl's Jr.	460	33	32	22	7	-	90	1110	2	6	-	0.25
1 ea.	Whopper	Burger King	678	53.9	31	37	12	1.48	87.3	910	5.24	12.2	-	0.16
1 ea.	Hamburger Famous Star	Carl's Jr.	580	49	25	32	9	-	70	910	2	10	-	0.3
	ZERO-VALUE													
1 ea.	Quarter Pounder w/cheese	McDonalds	513	39.7	29	28.3	11.2	1.69	93.5	1152	2.79	9.77	-	0.11
1 ea.	Double Western Bacon Cheeseburger	Carl's Jr.	900	64	51	49	21	-	155	1770	2	16	-	-
10 ea.	Chicken Nuggets	McDonald's	422	25.6	25.1	24.3	5.4	2.4	62.4	1118	0	0	-	-

MEAL: FAST FOODS (BURGER) GROUP: 41 CATEGORY: SIDE ITEMS

SELECTION TIPS: Baked potatoes are much better than fries. Small sizes are better than large. As always, watch for the amount of saturated fat.

Amt	Food	Brand	Kcal	CHO	PRO	FAT	Sat Fat	Trans Fat	Chol	Sodium	Fiber	Sugar	Fruit	Veggie
						GOLD								
1 ea.	Garden Salad w/o dressing	Wendy's	35	7	2	0	0	0	0	20	3	4	-	1.35
1 pk.	Salad Dressing, French, fat-free	Wendy's	90	21	0	0	0	0	0	240	1	18	-	-
1 ea.	Salad, Caesar, w/ chicken	McDonald's	100	3	17	2.5	1.5	-	40	240	2	1	-	0.57
1 ea.	Salad Dressing, vinaigrette, fat-free	McDonald's	35	8	0	0	0	0	0	260	0	6	-	-
						SILVER								
1 ea.	Nuts, almonds	Wendy's	130	4	4	12	1	0	0	70	2	1	-	-
1 ea.	Baked Potato	Wendy's	310	72	7	0	0	0	0	25	7	5	-	1.97
1 ea.	Chili, small	Wendy's	200	21	17	6	2.5	0	35	870	5	5	-	-
						BRONZE								
1 ea.	Taco Chips	Wendy's	220	25	3	11	2	2	0	150	2	0	-	-
1 ea.	French Fries, small	Burger King	230	26	2	13	3	3	0	380	2	-	-	0.9
1 ea.	Chili, large	Wendy's	300	31	25	9	3.5	0	50	1310	7	8	-	-
						ZERO-VALUE								
1 ea.	French Fries, large	McDonald's	576	70	5.7	30.5	6.09	8.06	0	331	7.01	0.29	-	1.71
1 ea.	Onion Rings, large	Carl's Jr.	430	53	7	21	5	-	0	700	3	7	-	0.73
1 ea.	Jalapeno Poppers	Burger King	230	22	7	13	5	-	20	790	2	1	-	0.16
1 ea.	Baked Potato, bacon & cheese	Wendy's	580	79	18	22	6	0	40	950	7	6	-	2.15

MEAL: FAST FOODS (BURGER)   GROUP: 42   CATEGORY: DESSERTS

SELECTION TIPS: Very few items are acceptable and most should be avoided. Breaking the habit of needing dessert is worth the effort. Watch carefully for high amounts of **calories** and **fat**. Remember that nothing taste better than thin feels.

Amt	Food	Brand	Kcal	CHO	PRO	FAT	Sat Fat	Trans Fat	Chol	Sodium	Fiber	Sugar	Fruit	Veggie
			GOLD - does not apply											
			SILVER - does not apply											
			BRONZE											
1 ea.	Fruit & Yogurt Parfait, w/o granola	McDonald's	128	25	3.5	1.6	0.01	0.08	7.1	54	1.3	17	0.37	-
1 ea.	Frozen Dessert, Coca-Cola	Burger King	370	92	0	0	0	0	0	-	0	92	-	-
1 ea.	Apple Dippers	McDonald's	98	23.2	0.4	0.69	0.37	0.01	2.67	35.6	-	15.3	-	-
1 ea.	Ice Cream Cone, vanilla, reduced fat	McDonald's	150	24	4	3.5	2	0	15	60	0	-	-	-
			ZERO-VALUE											
1 ea.	Sundae, hot fudge	McDonald's	333	54	7.4	10.6	6.4	0.43	23.2	168	0.72	48	-	-
1 ea.	Danish, apple	McDonald's	249	33.6	2.36	12	3.08	4.72	0	153	1.54	13.3	0.33	-
	Sweet Roll, cinnamon, w/o icing	Burger King	440	51	6	23	6	-	25	710	1	20	-	-
1 ea.	McFlurry, w/M&M's	McDonald's	620	96	14	20	12	1	55	190	1	-	-	-
1 ea.	Hershey's Sundaes Pie	Burger King	310	32	3	19	12	0	10	220	1	-	-	-
1 ea.	Frozen Dessert, medium	Wendy's	393	70.4	10.4	7.7	4.9	-	48	292	9.8	47	-	-
1 ea.	Milk Shake, small	Burger King	340	62	10	6	4	0	25	210	3	52	-	-
1 ea.	Milk Shake, medium	McDonald's	770	132	17.4	21.3	10.9	1.18	66	335	0.95	111	-	-
1 ea.	Triple Thick Shake, chocolate	McDonald's	1160	203	27	27	16	2	100	510	2	-	-	-

MEAL: FAST FOODS (NON-BURGER)   GROUP: 43   CATEGORY: BREAKFAST

SELECTION TIPS: It's difficult to find many healthy breakfast selections at a fast food establishment. The best you can do is a bagel or low fat muffin. You can also choose an egg dish without the sausage, bacon, or cheese.

Amt	Food	Brand	Kcal	CHO	PRO	FAT	Sat Fat	Trans Fat	Chol	Sodium	Fiber	Sugar	Fruit	Veggie
							GOLD - does not apply							
							SILVER							
1 ea.	Muffin, bran, low fat	Dunkin Donuts	260	59	4	1.5	0	-	0	440	4	33	-	-
							BRONZE							
1 ea.	Cheese & Egg on a Deli Roll	Subway	270	35	16	9	4	0	15	670	3	-	-	-
1 ea.	Bagel	Dunkin' Donuts	320	62	12	2.5	0.5	0	0	610	2	-	-	-
							ZERO-VALUE							
1 ea.	Glazed Doughnut	Arby's	200	22	2	12	3	4	5	95	<1	-	-	-
1 ea.	Steak & Cheese on a Deli Roll	Subway	490	37	30	26	10	0.5	65	1210	3	-	-	-
1 ea.	Biscuit w/sausage & gravy	Arby's	961	107	7	68	14	0	12	3755	1	-	-	-
1 ea.	Chocolate Chip Muffin	Dunkin' Donuts	630	89	10	26	8	0	70	560	2	-	-	-
1 ea.	Apple Fritter	Krispy Kreme	380	46	4	21	5	7	5	290	2	-	-	-
1 ea.	Blueberry Muffin	Arby's	320	49	4	12	2	0	20	490	1	-	-	-

MEAL: FAST FOODS (NON-BURGER)   GROUP: 44   CATEGORY: MAIN ITEMS

SELECTION TIPS: Common sense can go a long way when it comes to fast foods. First of all, do not make fast food a regular part of your diet. You may have good intentions, but sooner or later you will order something loaded with **calories** and **fat**. If you do your homework you will be able to find reasonably healthy choices at any fast food place. Don't forget to search the Internet (CalorieKing.com) for the best choices.

Amt	Food	Brand	Kcal	CHO	PRO	FAT	Sat Fat	Trans Fat	Chol	Sodium	Fiber	Sugar	Fruit	Veggie
						GOLD								
1 ea.	Chicken Soft Taco	Taco Bell	180	21	10	7	2	0.5	20	580	2	-	-	-
1 ea.	Turkey Sandwich, 6"	Subway	280	46	18	4.5	1.5	-	20	1010	4	5	-	0.16
1 ea.	Salad, Chicken Breast	Subway	120	14	12	2.5	0.5	0	20	59	4	-	-	-
1 ea.	Veggie-Delight, sandwich, 6""	Subway	230	44	9	3	1	-	0	510	4	5	-	0.17
						SILVER								
1 slice	Pizza, cheese, thin & crispy	Pizza Hut	200	21	10	8	4.5	0	25	570	1	-	-	-
1 ea.	Roast Beef, regular	Arby's	320	24	21	21	5	1	44	953	2	-	-	-
1 ea.	Caesar Salad, roasted chicken, w/o dressing	KFC	220	6	30	8	4.5	0	70	830	3	-	-	-
1 ea.	Tuna Sandwich, light mayonnaise, 6"	Subway	450	46	20	22	6	-	40	1190	4	5	-	-
						BRONZE								
1 ea.	Chicken Breast, original	KFC	380	11	40	19	6	-	145	1150	0	0	-	-
1 ea.	Meatball Sandwich, 6"	Subway	530	53	24	26	10	-	5.5	1360	6	7	-	-
						ZERO-VALUE								
1 ea.	Fiesta Taco Salad	Taco Bell	860	82	31	46	14	5	65	1800	12	-	-	-
1 ea.	Sandwich, roasted turkey ranch & bacon	Arby's	824	75	49	38	11	1	109	2258	5	-	-	-
1 ea.	Popcorn Chicken, large	KFC	560	31	29	36	7	3.5	35	1660	2	-	-	-
1 slice	Pizza, stuffed crust, supreme	Pizza Hut	410	42	20	18	8	0.5	50	1330	2	-	-	-

MEAL: FAST FOODS (NON-BURGER) GROUP: 45 CATEGORY: SIDE ITEMS

SELECTION TIPS: Baked potatoes are much better than fries. Small sizes are better than large. As always, watch for the amount of **saturated fat**.

Amt	Food	Brand	Kcal	CHO	PRO	FAT	Sat Fat	Trans Fat	Chol	Sodium	Fiber	Sugar	Fruit	Veggie
							GOLD							
1 ea.	Corn on the Cobb	KFC	70	13	2	1.5	0.5	0	0	5	3	-	-	1
1 ea.	Minestrone Soup	Subway	90	17	4	1	1	0	0	910	1	-	-	-
1 ea.	Green Beans	KFC	50	7	2	1.5	0	0	5	570	2	-	-	-
1 ea.	Baked Beans	KFC	220	45	8	1	0	0	5	730	7	-	-	-
							SILVER							
1 ea.	Mac & Cheese	KFC	130	15	5	6	2	-	5	610	1	1	-	-
1 ea.	Soup, Wild Rice w/chicken	Subway	230	26	6	11	3.5	0	50	1170	1	-	-	-
1 ea.	Mexican Rice	Taco Bell	200	26	6	9	3.5	0.5	15	850	2	-	-	-
1 ea.	Mashed Potatoes w/gravy	KFC	140	20	2	5	1	0.5	0	560	1	-	-	-
							BRONZE							
1 ea.	Pintos & Cheese	Taco Bell	180	20	10	7	3.5	1	15	700	6	-	-	-
1 ea.	Biscuit	KFC	220	24	4	11	2.5	3.5	0	640	1	-	-	-
							ZERO-VALUE							
1 ea.	Nachos, Bell Grande	Taco Bell	780	80	20	43	13	-	35	1300	12	6	-	-
1 ea.	Mozzarella Sticks	Arby's	426	38	18	28	13	2	45	1370	2	-	-	-
1 ea.	French Fries, large	Arby's	566	82	6	37	7	5	0	1029	6	-	-	1.3

MEAL: FAST FOODS (NON-BURGER)   GROUP: 46   CATEGORY: DESSERTS

SELECTION TIPS: Beware of the amount of **calories** and **fat**. Remember that nothing taste better than thin feels.

Amt	Food	Brand	Kcal	CHO	PRO	FAT	Sat Fat	Trans Fat	Chol	Sodium	Fiber	Sugar	Fruit	Veggie
							GOLD - does not apply							
							SILVER							
1 ea.	Fruizle, peach pizzazz	Subway	100	26	0	0	0	0	0	25	0	-	-	-
1 ea.	Fruizle, pineapple delight	Subway	160	40	1	0	0	0	0	25	2	-	0.2	-
							BRONZE							
1 slice	Apple Pie	KFC	280	44	2	11	2.5	2	0	230	2	-	-	-
1 ea.	Oatmeal Cookie, Sweet Lite	KFC	160	24	2	6	1.5	1	10	140	1	-	-	-
							ZERO-VALUE							
1 slice	Pecan Pie	KFC	480	67	5	21	4.5	1	40	360	12	6	-	-
1 ea.	Chocolate Chip Cookie	Subway	210	30	2	10	6	0	15	150	1	-	-	-
1 ea.	Fudge Brownie	KFC	280	43	3	11	4	0.5	20	200	1	-	-	-
1 ea.	Frozen Parfait, cherry cheesecake	KFC	300	46	3	11	5	-	4	130	2	37	-	-